Fluid and Electrolyte Therapy

Editors

ALLEN J. ROUSSEL
GEOF W. SMITH

VETERINARY CLINICS OF NORTH AMERICA: FOOD ANIMAL PRACTICE

www.vetfood.theclinics.com

Consulting Editor
ROBERT A. SMITH

July 2014 • Volume 30 • Number 2

ELSEVIER

1600 John F. Kennedy Boulevard • Suite 1800 • Philadelphia, Pennsylvania, 19103-2899

http://www.vetfood.theclinics.com

VETERINARY CLINICS OF NORTH AMERICA: FOOD ANIMAL PRACTICE Volume 30, Number 2
July 2014 ISSN 0749-0720, ISBN-13: 978-0-323-31175-5

Editor: Patrick Manley
Developmental Editor: Yonah Korngold

Veterinary Clinics of North America: Food Animal Practice (ISSN 0749-0720) is published in March, July, and November by Elsevier Inc., 360 Park Avenue South, New York, NY 10010-1710. Subscription prices are $235.00 per year (domestic individuals), $326.00 per year (domestic institutions), $110.00 per year (domestic students/residents), $265.00 per year (Canadian individuals), $430.00 per year (Canadian institutions), $335.00 per year (international individuals), $430.00 per year (international institutions), and $165.00 per year (international and Canadian students/residents). To receive student/resident rate, orders must be accompanied by name of affiliated institution, date of term, and the signature of program/residency coordinator on institution letterhead. *Clinics* subscription prices. All prices are subject to change without notice. **POSTMASTER:** Send address changes to *Veterinary Clinics of North America: Food Animal Practice*, Elsevier Health Sciences Division, Subscription Customer Service, 3251 Riverport Lane, Maryland Heights, MO 63043. Customer Service (orders, claims, online, change of address): Elsevier Health Sciences Division, Subscription Customer Service, 3251 Riverport Lane, Maryland Heights, MO 63043. Tel: 1-800-654-2452 (U.S. and Canada); 314-447-8871 (ouside U.S. and Canada). Fax: 314-447-8029. E-mail: journalscustomerservice-usa@elsevier.com (for print support); journalsonlinesupport-usa@elsevier.com (for online support).

Reprints. For copies of 100 or more, of articles in this publication, please contact the Commercial Reprints Department, Elsevier Inc., 360 Park Avenue South, New York, NY 10010-1710. Tel.: 212-633-3874; Fax: 212-633-3820; E-mail: reprints@elsevier.com.

Veterinary Clinics of North America: Food Animal Practice is covered in *Current Contents/Agriculture, Biology and Environmental Sciences, MEDLINE/PubMed (Index Medicus), and Excerpta Medica.*

Contributors

CONSULTING EDITOR

ROBERT A. SMITH, DVM, MS
Diplomate, American Board of Veterinary Practitioners; Veterinary Research and Consulting Services, LLC, Greeley, Colorado

EDITORS

ALLEN J. ROUSSEL, DVM, MS
Diplomate, European College of Bovine Health Management; Diplomate, American College of Veterinary Internal Medicine; Professor and Head, Department of Large Animal Clinical Sciences, College of Veterinary Medicine and Biomedical Sciences, Texas A&M University, College Station, Texas

GEOF W. SMITH, DVM, MS, PhD
Diplomate, American College of Veterinary Internal Medicine; Professor of Ruminant Medicine, Department of Population Health and Pathobiology, College of Veterinary Medicine, North Carolina State University, Raleigh, North Carolina

AUTHORS

CHRISTIE BALCOMB, BVSc
William R. Pritchard Veterinary Medical Teaching Hospital, University of California, Davis, Davis California

JOACHIM BERCHTOLD, Dr Med Vet
Diplomate, European College of Bovine Health Management; Veterinary Specialist for Cattle, Tierärztliche Praxis Dr. Berchtold, Pittenhart, Germany

STACEY R. BYERS, DVM, MS
Diplomate, American College of Veterinary Internal Medicine; Department of Clinical Sciences, College of Veterinary Medicine and Biomedical Sciences, Colorado State University, Fort Collins, Colorado

PETER D. CONSTABLE, BVSc(Hons), MS, PhD, MRCVS
Diplomate, American College of Veterinary Internal Medicine; Diplomate, American College of Veterinary Nutrition (Honorary); Dean, Department of Veterinary Clinical Medicine, College of Veterinary Medicine, University of Illinois at Urbana-Champaign, Urbana, Illinois

GILLES FECTEAU
Diplomate, American College of Veterinary Internal Medicine; Professor of Bovine Medicine, Département de Sciences Cliniques, Faculté de Médecine Vétérinaire, Université de Montréal, Saint-Hyacinthe, Québec, Canada

DEREK FOSTER, DVM, PhD
Department of Population Health and Pathobiology, College of Veterinary Medicine, North Carolina State University, Raleigh, North Carolina

ARCANGELO GENTILE, Dr med vet
Department of Veterinary Medical Sciences, University of Bologna, Ozzano Emilia, Bologna, Italy

JESSE P. GOFF, DVM, PhD
Professor, Department of Biomedical Sciences, College of Veterinary Medicine, Iowa State University, Ames, Iowa

WALTER GRÜNBERG, Dr med vet, MS, PhD
Diplomate, European College of Bovine Health Managament; Diplomate, European College of Animal Reproduction; Clinic for Cattle, University of Veterinary Medicine Hannover, Foundation, Hanover, Germany

MEREDYTH JONES, DVM, MS
Diplomate, American College of Veterinary Internal Medicine; Assistant Professor, Food Animal Field Services, Department of Large Animal Clinical Sciences, College of Veterinary Medicine, Texas A&M University, College Station, Texas

ANDREA S. LEAR, DVM
Department of Clinical Sciences, College of Veterinary Medicine and Biomedical Sciences, Colorado State University, Fort Collins, Colorado

INGRID LORENZ, Dr med vet, Dr med vet habil
UCD School of Veterinary Medicine, University College Dublin, Belfield, Dublin, Ireland

CHRISTINE NAVARRE, DVM, MS
Diplomate, American College of Veterinary Internal Medicine; LSU AgCenter, Baton Rouge, Louisiana

ALLEN J. ROUSSEL, DVM, MS
Diplomate, European College of Bovine Health Management; Diplomate, American College of Veterinary Internal Medicine; Professor and Head, Department of Large Animal Clinical Sciences, College of Veterinary Medicine and Biomedical Sciences, Texas A&M University, Texas

NICOLAS SATTLER
Diplomate, American College of Veterinary Internal Medicine; Bovine Practitioners, Clinique Vétérinaire St-Vallier, Saint-Vallier, Québec, Canada

GEOF W. SMITH, DVM, MS, PhD
Diplomate, American College of Veterinary Internal Medicine; Professor of Ruminant Medicine, Department of Population Health and Pathobiology, College of Veterinary Medicine, North Carolina State University, Raleigh, North Carolina

DAVID C. VAN METRE, DVM
Diplomate, American College of Veterinary Internal Medicine; Department of Clinical Sciences, College of Veterinary Medicine and Biomedical Sciences, Colorado State University, Fort Collins, Colorado

Contents

At present, except for animals treated with repeated isoflupredone acetate administration, the exact determinants causing hypokalemia syndrome remain uncertain. Affected animals are anorexic, weak to recumbent, and most often show signs of gastrointestinal stasis. Treatment is directed toward supportive care and oral potassium supplementation.

Hypocalcemia is a clinical disorder that can be life threatening to the cow (milk fever) and predisposes the animal to various other metabolic and infectious disorders. Calcium homeostasis is mediated primarily by parathyroid hormone, which stimulates bone calcium resorption and renal calcium reabsorption. Parathyroid hormone stimulates the production of 1,25-dihydroxyvitamin D to enhance diet calcium absorption. High dietary cation-anion difference interferes with tissue sensitivity to parathyroid hormone. Hypomagnesemia reduces tissue response to parathyroid hormone.

Phosphorus (P) homeostasis in ruminants has received increased attention over the past decades. Although environmental concerns associated with excessive P excretion in cattle manure have led to incentives to lower dietary P intake, hypophosphatemia—particularly in the periparturient dairy cow—has been associated with conditions, such as the downer cow syndrome or postparturient hemoglobinuria. The objective of this article is to revisit current understanding of P homeostasis in ruminants, to discuss the pathophysiology and clinical presentation of P balance disorders, and to review different treatment approaches to correct imbalances of the body's P equilibrium.

Early and aggressive fluid therapy is critical in correcting the metabolic complications associated with calf diarrhea. Oral electrolyte therapy can be used with success in calves, but careful consideration should be given to the type of oral electrolyte used. Electrolyte solutions with high osmolalities can significantly slow abomasal emptying and can be a risk factor for abomasal bloat in calves. Milk should not be withheld from calves with diarrhea for more than 12 to 24 hours. Hypertonic saline and hypertonic sodium bicarbonate can be used effectively for intravenous fluid therapy on farms when intravenous catheterization is not possible.

Fluid therapy for mature cattle differs from that for calves because the common conditions that result in dehydration and the metabolic derangements that accompany these conditions are different. The veterinarian needs to know which problem exists, what to administer to correct the problem, in what quantity, by what route, and at what rate. Mature cattle more frequently suffer from alkalosis; therefore, acidifying solutions containing K^+ and Cl^- in concentrations greater than that of plasma are frequently indicated. The rumen provides a large-capacity reservoir into which oral rehydration solutions may be administered, which can save time and money.

Body water, electrolytes, and acid-base balance are important consider-ations in the evaluation and treatment of small ruminants and camelids with any disease process, with restoration of these a priority as adjunctive therapy. The goals of fluid therapy should be to maintain cardiac output and tissue perfusion, and to correct acid-base and electrolyte abnormalities. Hypoglycemia, hyperkalemia, and acidosis are the most life-threatening abnormalities, and require most immediate correction.

The use of whole blood and/or blood products is indicated in ruminant medicine. The goal of this article is to summarize previous literature on blood groups in ruminants and camelids, list indications for transfusion, and describe collection and transfusion techniques applicable to small ruminants and cattle that can be used in practice.

VETERINARY CLINICS OF NORTH AMERICA: FOOD ANIMAL PRACTICE

Preface

Fluid and Electrolyte Therapy

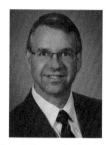 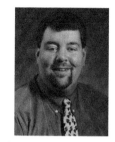

Allen J. Roussel, DVM, MS   Geof W. Smith, DVM, MS, PhD
Editors

It has been 15 years since the previous issue of "Fluid and Electrolyte Therapy" was published in the November 1999 *Veterinary Clinics of North America: Food Animal Practice*. However, fluid therapy still plays a critical role in ruminant medicine. In this issue, we have tried to provide veterinarians with practical information on fluid and electrolyte therapy that can be easily incorporated into all types of practices. There are articles on fairly complex subjects, such as the pathophysiology of acid-base abnormalities and the application of strong ion and Henderson-Hasselbalch theories to common ruminant diseases, as well as a detailed article on D-lactic acidosis in calves. There are also articles on disturbances of electrolytes in ruminants, including calcium, magnesium, potassium, phosphorus, and sodium. Additional articles provide specific fluid therapy recommendations for both neonatal and adult cattle, as well as small ruminants and camelids.

This issue of the *Veterinary Clinics of North America: Food Animal Practice* was written by ruminant clinicians for the practicing veterinarian. Due to the large size of ruminants and the economics of food animal agriculture, fluid therapy is often seen as difficult to accomplish in practice. However, there are clinical situations where aggressive fluid therapy can be done quite easily and can dramatically improve the clinical outcome. The authors in this issue represent six countries and bring a broad collection of knowledge and experiences that should be of use to all ruminant veterinarians. Many advances in our understanding of fluid and electrolyte therapy have been made in the past 15 years since the original issue was published, and we have attempted to incorporate current information into each article.

Vet Clin Food Anim 30 (2014) ix–x
http://dx.doi.org/10.1016/j.cvfa.2014.05.001
0749-0720/14/$ – see front matter © 2014 Published by Elsevier Inc.

vetfood.theclinics.com

We would like to extend our sincere thanks to all the authors for agreeing to partic-ipate in this project, and for sharing their knowledge and clinical experience. We hope that this issue proves to be a useful reference for practitioners in the field.

Allen J. Roussel, DVM, MS
Department of Large Animal Clinical Sciences
College of Veterinary Medicine
Texas A&M University
College Station, TX 77843-4475, USA

Geof W. Smith, DVM, MS, PhD
Department of Population Health and Pathobiology
College of Veterinary Medicine
North Carolina State University
1060 William Moore Drive
Raleigh, NC 27607, USA

E-mail addresses:
ARoussel@cvm.tamu.edu (A.J. Roussel)
Geoffrey_Smith@ncsu.edu (G.W. Smith)

Acid-Base Assessment

When and How To Apply the Henderson-Hasselbalch Equation and Strong Ion Difference Theory

Peter D. Constable, MS, PhD, MRCVS

KEYWORDS

- Acidosis • Alkalosis • Total CO_2 • Anion gap • Strong ion gap

KEY POINTS

- The Henderson-Hasselbalch equation is probably the most famous equation in biology but is more descriptive than mechanistic.
- The traditional approach to acid-base assessment using the Henderson-Hasselbalch equation provides a clinically useful and accurate method when plasma protein concentrations are within the reference range.
- The Henderson-Hasselbalch equation cannot explain why abnormal plasma protein concentrations change plasma pH, why ingestion of $CaCl_2$ is acidifying, and why the rapid intravenous administration of large volume 0.9% NaCl solution is acidifying.
- The Henderson-Hasselbalch equation is a simplified version of strong ion difference (SID) theory that assumes plasma protein concentration is fixed within the reference range.
- The simplified strong ion approach is a mechanistic acid-base model that can provide new insight into complicated acid-base disturbances.
- The simplified strong ion approach should be used to evaluate acid-base balance whenever plasma protein concentrations are abnormal.

A revolution is under way in the clinical assessment of acid-base status. All veterinarians are familiar with the Henderson-Hasselbalch equation, which was formulated in 1916.[1,2] Clinically important applications of the equation include development of the base excess (BE) concept by Astrup and colleagues in 1960[3,4] and introduction of the anion gap (AG) concept in the 1970s and 1980s.[5,6] Application of the Henderson-Hasselbalch equation has greatly facilitated the diagnosis and treatment of acid-base and electrolyte abnormalities in humans and domestic animals.

The author has nothing to disclose.
College of Veterinary Medicine, University of Illinois at Urbana-Champaign, 2001 South Lincoln Avenue, Urbana, IL 61802, USA
E-mail address: constabl@illinois.edu

Vet Clin Food Anim 30 (2014) 295–316
http://dx.doi.org/10.1016/j.cvfa.2014.03.001   **vetfood.theclinics.com**

Two quantitative mechanistic physicochemical approaches have been developed to describe acid-base balance in animals[7]: Stewart's strong ion model[8–10] and Constable's simplified strong ion model.[11] The 2 strong ion approaches use a systems approach that makes a clear conceptual distinction between dependent and independent variables. In this context, independent variables influence a system from the outside and cannot be affected by changes within the system or by changes in other independent variables. In contrast, dependent variables are influenced directly and predictably by changes in the independent variables.

The purpose of this brief review is to summarize the key concepts in the Henderson-Hasselbalch equation and SID approach, identify existing anomalies with the Henderson-Hasselbalch equation, demonstrate how the Henderson-Hasselbalch equation is a simplification of SID theory, and provide clinically relevant guidelines for the evaluation of acid-base balance in neonatal calves and adult cattle. Additional reviews can be consulted if more detailed information is required regarding acid-base assessment using the Henderson-Hasselbalch equation or SID approach in cattle.[12–16]

THE HENDERSON-HASSELBALCH EQUATION

The traditional approach for assessing acid-base balance in animals uses the Henderson-Hasselbalch equations and focuses on how plasma pH is determined by the interaction between carbon dioxide tension (P_{CO_2}), the bicarbonate concentration ($cHCO_3^-$), the negative logarithm of the apparent dissociation constant (pK_1') for carbonic acid (H_2CO_3), and the solubility coefficient for CO_2 in plasma (S). The dissociation equilibrium of carbonic acid can be represented by[1,2]

$$P_{CO_2} \leftrightarrow CO_2(aq) + H_2O \leftrightarrow H_2CO_3 \leftrightarrow H^+ + HCO_3^- \tag{1}$$

where $CO_2(aq)$ is dissolved CO_2.

The equilibrium reaction of carbonic acid is most commonly expressed as the Henderson-Hasselbalch equation:

$$pH = pK_1' + \log_{10}\{cHCO_3^-/(S \cdot P_{CO_2})\} \tag{2}$$

with the recommended value for pK_1' in human blood at 37°C and an ionic strength of 0.16 mol/L (mammalian extracellular fluid) 6.105 and S 0.0307 [mmol/L]/mm Hg. The evaluation of acid-base balance using the Henderson-Hasselbalch equation uses pH as an overall measure of acid-base status, P_{CO_2} as an independent measure of the respiratory component of acid-base balance, and plasma $cHCO_3^-$ or BE as a measure of the metabolic (nonrespiratory) component of acid-base balance (**Fig. 1**).[13]

The actual $cHCO_3^-$ (in units of mmol/L) is calculated using the Henderson-Hasselbalch equation, measured values for pH and P_{CO_2}, and documented values for pK_1' and S for blood, whereby[17–19]

$$cHCO_3^- = S \times P_{CO_2} \times 10^{(pH - pK1')} = 0.0307 \times P_{CO_2} \times 10^{(pH - 6.105)} \tag{3}$$

This equation assumes a fixed and constant value for pK_1'; this assumption has been questioned when Equation (3) was applied to blood from critically ill patients with varying sodium and plasma protein concentrations.[20,21]

BE is calculated from the results of routine blood gas and pH analysis using the van Slyke equation with hemoglobin concentration ([Hb]) and $cHCO_3^-$ in mmol/L[22]:

$$BE = (1 - 0.023 \times [Hb]) \times \{cHCO_3^- - 24.4 + (7.7 + 2.3 \times [Hb]) \times (pH - 7.40)\} \tag{4}$$

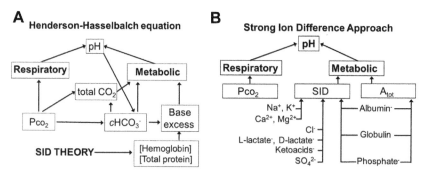

Fig. 1. Evaluation of acid-base balance using the traditional Henderson-Hasselbalch equation (*A*) and SID theory (*B*). The Henderson-Hasslebalch equation posits that blood pH is dependent on the respiratory system, as assessed by the P_{CO_2}, and metabolism, as assessed by the $cHCO_3^-$ or BE. Image *A* highlights one of the fundamental flaws with using the Henderson-Hasselbalch equation in that blood pH cannot be dependent on $cHCO_3^-$ because $cHCO_3^-$ is calculated from blood pH and P_{CO_2}. For comparison, the strong ion approach to acid-base balance posits that blood pH is dependent on the respiratory system, assessed by P_{CO_2}, and on metabolism, assessed by the SID and concentration of nonvolatile buffers (A_{tot}, such as albumin, globulin, and phosphate) in plasma. (*Adapted from* Constable PD. Clinical assessment of acid-base status: Strong ion difference theory. Vet Clin North Am Food Anim Pract 1999;15:447–71.)

Standardized BE (SBE), which is also called the extracellular fluid BE (BEecf), is calculated assuming [Hb] = 3.1 mmol/L = 5 g/dL[19]:

$$SBE = BEecf = 0.93 \times \{cHCO_3^- - 24.4 + 14.83 \times (pH - 7.40)\} \tag{5}$$

The SBE is easy to calculate from the results of blood gas and pH analysis and indicates the direction and magnitude of an acid-base disturbance. SBE does not, however, provide insight into the mechanism for the acid-base disturbance.[23]

The Henderson-Hasselbalch equation has proved helpful in facilitating understanding of mammalian acid-base physiology and is routinely used in the treatment of acid-base abnormalities. With use of the traditional Henderson-Hasselbalch equation, 4 primary acid-base disturbances have been defined[24]: respiratory acidosis (increased P_{CO_2}), respiratory alkalosis (decreased P_{CO_2}), metabolic acidosis (decreased $cHCO_3^-$ or BE), and metabolic alkalosis (increased $cHCO_3^-$ or BE) (**Box 1, Fig. 2**).

Some blood gas analyzers calculate plasma $cHCO_3^-$ using a value of 6.10 or 6.095 for pK_1' instead of the recommended value of 6.105 when analyzing a blood sample.[19] Some blood gas analyzers also calculate BE and SBE (BEecf) using equations different from those presented in Equations (4) and (5), meaning that reported values differ despite identical values for pH, P_{CO_2}, and [Hb].[25,26] Accurate calculation of BE and SBE assumes that the plasma protein concentration is within the reference range, which is often not the case in critically ill animals.

At least 3 clinically important anomalies have been identified when the Henderson-Hasselbalch equation is applied to acid-base abnormalities. First, the Henderson-Hasselbalch equation does not provide an explanation as to why an abnormal plasma protein concentration alters pH. Second, the equation does not explain why ingestion of $CaCl_2$ by adult cattle is acidifying. Third, the equation does not explain why the rapid intravenous administration of 0.9% NaCl, Na-gluconate, 5% dextrose, or Ringer solution is acidifying. Anomalies are helpful in identifying inadequacies of an old model and

> **Box 1**
> **Recommended methods to diagnose acid-base disturbances in neonatal calves and adult cattle**
>
> 1. **Routine screening test** (measure 1 parameter: $ctCO_2$ in plasma or serum)
>
> | | Metabolic (Nonrespiratory) |
> | --- | --- |
> | | Abnormal total CO_2 |
> | Acidosis | ↓ $ctCO_2$ |
> | Alkalosis | ↑ $ctCO_2$ |
>
> 2. **If total protein concentration is approximately normal, then apply the Henderson-Hasselbalch equation** (measure 5 parameters: pH, P_{CO_2}, $[Na^+]$, $[K^+]$, and $[Cl^-]$; and calculate BE, the $cHCO_3^-$, and the AG from these measurements). The AG is calculated to determine if unmeasured anions are present.
>
> | | Respiratory | Metabolic (Nonrespiratory) |
> | --- | --- | --- |
> | | Abnormal P_{CO_2} | Abnormal extracellular BE (SBE or BEecf) |
> | Acidosis | ↑P_{CO_2} | ↓ BE (preferred) or ↓ $cHCO_3^-$ |
> | Alkalosis | ↓P_{CO_2} | ↑ BE (preferred) or ↑ $cHCO_3^-$ |
>
> Unmeasured anions present: ↑ anion gap
>
> 3. **If total protein concentration is abnormal, then apply the simplified strong ion approach** (measure 6 parameters: pH, P_{CO_2}, $[Na^+]$, $[K^+]$, $[Cl^-]$, and [total protein]). The SIG is calculated to determine if unmeasured strong ions are present.
>
> | | Respiratory | Metabolic (Nonrespiratory) | |
> | --- | --- | --- | --- |
> | | Abnormal P_{CO_2} | Abnormal SID | Abnormal A_{tot} |
> | Acidosis | ↑P_{CO_2} | ↓ SID | ↑ [Total protein] |
> | Alkalosis | ↓ P_{CO_2} | ↑ SID | ↓ [Total protein] |
>
> Unmeasured strong anions present: ↓ SIG (more negative)
>   Venous blood samples should be used unless respiratory disease is present, in which case arterial blood samples should be obtained.
>
> *Adapted from* Constable PD. Clinical assessment of acid-base status: strong ion difference theory. Vet Clin North Am Food Anim Pract 1999;15:447–71.

emphasizing the merits of a new model.[27] Of relevance to this discussion is that the simplified SID model for acid-base equilibrium provides a satisfactory explanation for all 3 anomalies.

THE STRONG ION DIFFERENCE APPROACH

Stewart proposed that plasma pH was determined by 3 independent factors: P_{CO_2}; the SID, which is the difference between the charge of plasma strong cations (sodium, potassium, calcium, and magnesium) and anions (chloride, lactate, sulfate, ketoacids, nonesterified fatty acids, and many others), in which strong cations and anions are fully dissociated at physiologic pH; and A_{tot}, which is the total plasma concentration of nonvolatile buffers (albumin, globulins, and inorganic phosphate).[8–10] In this context, pH and $cHCO_3^-$ are dependent variables, and 3 independent variables (SID, P_{CO_2}, and plasma nonvolatile buffer ion concentration) directly determine plasma pH (see **Fig. 1**).

From the 3 independent factors (P_{CO_2}, SID, and A_{tot}), Stewart developed a complicated polynomial equation that expressed pH (he erroneously used hydrogen ion concentration instead of hydrogen ion activity) as a function of 8 factors,

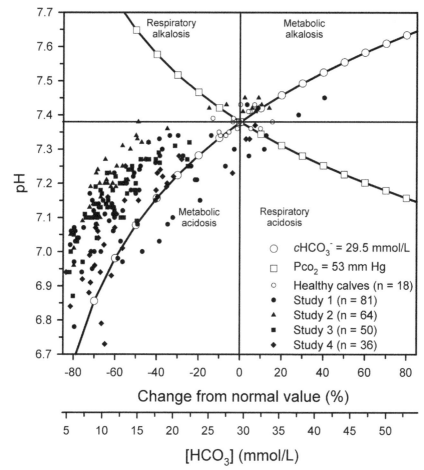

Fig. 2. Spider plot reveals the association between changes in 2 variables of the Henderson-Hasselbalch equation, plasma $cHCO_3^-$ and carbon dioxide tension (PCO_2), on venous blood pH in 231 sick calves, most of which had diarrhea. The spider plot was obtained by systematically varying one input variable ($cHCO_3^-$ or PCO_2) while holding the remaining input variables at their reference values for calf venous plasma. Reference values for the 2 input variables for calf plasma were 29.5 mmol/L for $cHCO_3^-$ (*large open circle*) and 53 mm Hg for PCO_2 (*open square*). The solid vertical and horizontal lines indicate that venous blood pH = 7.38 when $cHCO_3^-$ and PCO_2 are at their reference values. Note that the individual data points are displaced from the predicted pH–$cHCO_3^-$ relationship. This displacement indicates that changes in plasma $cHCO_3^-$ do not account for all of the changes in blood pH in sick calves.

consisting of 3 independent factors and 5 constants.[9,10] Constable subsequently showed algebraically[11] and graphically[28] that changes in 2 of Stewart's 8 factors had no quantitative effect on pH, resulting in the development of the 6-factor simplified strong ion equation (see **Fig. 1**). Currently, Constable's 6-factor simplified strong ion equation is the preferred form for applying the strong ion approach[11,13]; the equation states that pH is a function of 3 independent factors (PCO_2, SID, and A_{tot}) and 3 constants (S, the apparent dissociation constant for plasma carbonic acid [K_1'], and Ka, the effective dissociation constant for nonvolatile buffers in plasma), such that

$$pH = \log_{10}(2SID/[K_1'S\ Pco_2 + K_aA_{tot} - K_aSID + \sqrt{\{(K_1'S\ Pco_2 + K_aSID + K_aA_{tot})^2}$$
$$- 4K_a^2SIDA_{tot}\}])\tag{6}$$

The strong ion approach requires species-specific values for the total plasma concentration of nonvolatile weak acids (A_{tot}) in mmol/L and the effective dissociation constant (K_a) for plasma nonvolatile buffers. Values for A_{tot} (0.343 × [total protein, g/L] or 0.622 × [albumin, g/L]); K_a (0.8 × 10^{-7}; pK_a = 7.08) have been experimentally determined for calf plasma,[29] and similar values have been theoretically determined for plasma from adult cattle.[30] These experimentally determined values should be used whenever SID theory is applied to adult cattle or calves.

Several clinical ramifications arise from the simplified strong ion equation (Equation 6). Because clinically important acid-base derangements result from changes in Pco_2, SID, or concentrations of individual nonvolatile plasma buffers (A_{tot}; albumin, globulins, and phosphate), the strong ion approach distinguishes 6 primary acid-base disturbances (respiratory, strong ion, or nonvolatile buffer ion acidosis and alkalosis [**Fig. 3**]).[10,11] Acidemia results from an increase in Pco_2 and nonvolatile buffer concentrations (albumin, globulin, and phosphate) or from a decrease in SID. Alkalemia results from a decrease in Pco_2 and nonvolatile buffer concentration or from an increase in SID (see **Box 1, Fig. 3**). The 6 primary acid-base disturbances identified by SID theory (see **Figs. 1** and **3**) should be compared with the 4 primary acid-base disturbances identified by the Henderson-Hasselbalch equation (see **Figs. 1** and **2**).

The strong ion model offers a novel insight into the pathophysiology of mixed acid-base disorders and is mechanistic. The change in SID from normal is equivalent to the BE value, assuming a normal nonvolatile buffer ion concentration (normal albumin, globulins, and phosphate concentrations). This means that clinicians who have used the traditional Henderson-Hasselbalch approach with BE to indicate the metabolic component of the derangement have unknowingly been using the strong ion approach to evaluate acid-base status, because albumin, globulin, and phosphate concentrations are often normal. The strong ion model also explains how hypoproteinemia and hyperproteinemia alter pH (through alterations in A_{tot}), whereas the Henderson-Hasselbalch equation provides no such explanation.

An important and underappreciated aspect of the simplified strong ion equation is that it simplifies to the Henderson-Hasselbalch equation when applied to aqueous nonprotein solutions. This is understood most easily by algebraic rearrangement of the simplified strong ion equation (Equation 6), providing[11]

$$pH = pK_1' + \log\{SID - [A_{tot}/(1 + 10^{pKa\ -\ pH})]\}/(S\ Pco_2)\tag{7}$$

In aqueous nonprotein solutions, A_{tot} = 0 mEq/L and, therefore, Equation (7) is equivalent to[1,2]

$$pH = pK_1' + \log\{SID\}/(S\ Pco_2)\tag{8}$$

Comparison of Equation 8 to the Henderson-Hasselbalch equation (Equation 2) indicates that SID theory produces a general equation for clinical acid-base equilibrium in nonprotein solutions (where $cHCO_3^- = SID$). The simplified strong ion model, therefore, unites the Henderson-Hasselbalch equation and Stewart's strong ion model when applied to protein and phosphate-free solutions. Clinicians who ignore SID theory but enthusiastically embrace the Henderson-Hasselbalch equation when

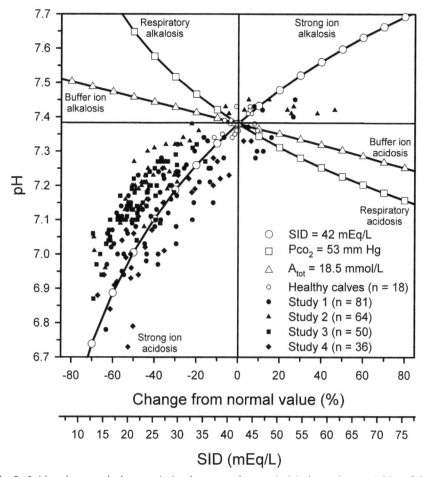

Fig. 3. Spider plot reveals the association between changes in 3 independent variables of the simplified strong ion equation, SID (*open circle*), carbon dioxide tension (Pco$_2$ [*open square*]), and the plasma concentration of nonvolatile buffers (Atot [*open triangle*]), on venous blood pH in 231 sick calves, most of which had diarrhea. The spider plot was obtained by systematically varying 1 input variable (SID, Pco$_2$, or Atot) while holding the remaining input variables at their reference values for calf venous plasma (42 mEq/L for SID), 53 mm Hg for Pco$_2$, and 18.5 mmol/L for Atot. The solid vertical and horizontal lines indicate that venous blood pH = 7.38 when SID, Pco$_2$, and Atot are at their reference values. Note that the individual data points are located more centrally around the predicted pH-SID relationship than for the pH-cHCO$_3^-$ relationship identified in **Fig. 2**. This is because changes in plasma protein concentration (and therefore Atot) due to changes in hydration status account for some of the change in blood pH. The plot also indicates the 6 primary acid-base disturbances (respiratory, strong ion, or nonvolatile buffer ion acidosis and alkalosis) and the relative effect of each disturbance on blood pH in the neonatal calf. Note that changes in SID have the greatest relative effect on blood pH. (*Adapted from* Constable PD, Stämpfli HR, Navetat H, et al. Use of a quantitative strong ion approach to determine the mechanism for acid-base abnormalities in sick calves with or without diarrhea. J Vet Intern Med 2005;19:581–9.)

diagnosing and treating acid-base imbalances need to recognize that they are using a simplified version of SID theory. The Henderson-Hasselbalch and SID approaches are not mutually exclusive; they effectively are the same approach in nonprotein-containing aqueous solutions but differ in their approach in protein-containing solutions, such as plasma.

THREE ANOMALIES OF THE HENDERSON-HASSELBALCH EQUATION
Failure to Explain Why an Abnormal Plasma Protein Concentration Changes Plasma pH

van Slyke,[31] in 1928, identified that plasma proteins play a role in acid-base balance. Subsequent experimental studies have conclusively shown that changes in plasma protein concentration cause plasma pH to change.[3,32–34] The Henderson-Hasselbalch equation (Equation 2) does not provide an explanation for this phenomenon. Although the total concentration of weak acids (A_{tot}) is not regulated to ensure acid-base homeostasis,[33] changes in A_{tot} have a direct and independent effect on plasma pH.[32,33] The form of the simplified strong ion equation provided in Equation (7) provides a clear mechanism for the effect of plasma protein concentration on pH, in that change in the plasma protein concentration has a direct effect on A_{tot} which leads to a direct and predictable change in plasma pH. Decreasing the plasma albumin concentration (thereby decreasing the concentration of nonvolatile buffers) increases plasma pH (see **Fig. 3**). Conversely, increasing the plasma albumin concentration (thereby increasing the concentration of nonvolatile buffers) decreases plasma pH.[33]

Failure to Explain Why Ingestion of $CaCl_2$ Is Acidifying

The mineral content of a diet can have a great influence on the incidence of milk fever in dairy cattle. Diets fed to dry cows typically have a greater concentration of strong cations (such as Na^+ and K^+) than anions (such as Cl^- and SO_4^{2-}). If the strong cations are absorbed from the intestinal tract to a greater extent than strong anions, the typical dry cow diet increases plasma SID, thereby creating a strong ion alkalosis (metabolic alkalosis). The normal forage-based dry cow diet is, therefore, called alkalogenic or cationic. The most widely used formula to characterize dietary cation-anion difference (DCAD) of cattle diets is[35]

$$DCAD = ([Na^+] + [K^+]) - ([Cl^-] + [SO_4^{2-}]) \tag{9}$$

The DCAD of a typical dry cow diet is +50 to +300 mEq/kg of dry matter (+5 to +30 mEq/100 g of dry matter); the plus sign indicates that strong cation concentration exceeds the strong anion concentration.

Feeding an acidogenic dry cow diet (DCAD −150 to 0 mEq/kg dry matter, equivalent to −15 to 0 mEq/100 g of dry matter) provides an effective method for decreasing the incidence of clinical hypocalcemia in periparturient dairy cows. Acidogenic salts produce a variable effect on mean 24-hour blood pH in nonlactating cattle when fed on the same molar basis (2 Eq/d), such as control (blood pH = 7.38, urine pH = 7.99), $CaCl_2$ (blood pH = 7.34, urine pH = 6.47), NH_4Cl (blood pH = 7.35, urine pH = 6.78), $MgCl_2$ (blood pH = 7.35, urine pH = 6.87), $CaSO_4$ (blood pH = 7.36, urine pH = 7.03), $(NH_4)_2SO_4$ (blood pH = 7.36, urine pH = 7.22), and $MgSO_4$ (blood pH = 7.37, urine pH = 7.41).[36] The Henderson-Hasselbalch equation provides no explanation for the differing effect of acidogenic salts on blood pH and urine pH and cannot provide a satisfactory explanation as to why $CaCl_2$ is acidifying when ingested. In contrast, SID theory posits that ingestion of acidogenic salts induces a systemic strong ion acidosis (metabolic acidosis) because of differential absorption of strong cations and anions from the intestinal tract, in that strong anions, such as Cl^- and SO_4^{2-}, are absorbed to a greater extent than strong cations, such as Ca^{2+} and NH_4^+, leading to a decrease in plasma SID and strong ion acidosis.

Failure to Explain Why the Rapid Intravenous Administration of Large Volume 0.9% NaCl Solution Is Acidifying

The rapid infusion of 0.9% NaCl solution produces a predictable, dose-dependent acidemia and metabolic acidosis characterized by hyperchloremia and a decreased plasma $cHCO_3^-$.[37,38] The phenomenon is called hyperchloremic acidosis and has been observed for more than 6 decades.[37,39] The Henderson-Hasselbalch equation fails to provide an adequate explanation for this phenomenon.

The traditional Henderson-Hasselbalch (bicarbonate-centered) view of acid-base equilibrium states that rapid infusion of large volumes of 0.9% NaCl solution creates a metabolic acidosis primarily by decreasing plasma $cHCO_3^-$ (and, therefore, pH as indicated by Equation 2) by increasing the distribution volume for bicarbonate without changing Pco_2. Application of the Henderson-Hasselbalch equation (Equation 2) to the normal values for human blood (pH, 7.40; Pco_2, 40 mm Hg; pK_1', 6.105; and S, 0.0307 [mmol/L]/mm Hg) produces a calculated plasma $cHCO_3^-$ of approximately 24 mmol/L. Accordingly, the bicarbonate-centered argument is that rapid intravenous infusion of large volumes of a solution with an effective $cHCO_3^-$ greater than 24 mmol/L increases plasma $cHCO_3^-$ and induces metabolic alkalosis, whereas infusion of a solution with a $cHCO_3^-$ less than 24 mmol/L (such as 0.9% NaCl or isotonic sodium gluconate where $cHCO_3^- = 0$ mmol/L) decreases plasma $cHCO_3^-$ and creates a metabolic acidosis and acidemia (see **Fig. 2**).[29] This mechanism is termed, *dilutional acidosis*. The dilutional acidosis explanation is so seductively simple that a majority of clinicians have not been interested in pursuing other, more likely, mechanisms for the development of metabolic acidosis.[40,41] Dilutional acidosis, however, is fundamentally flawed as an explanation for hyperchloremic acidosis because Equation 2 indicates that simple dilution must equally dilute all plasma acids (such as carbonic acid and, therefore, the value for $S \cdot Pco_2$) and bases (such as $cHCO_3^-$) and not cause a preferential decrease in plasma $cHCO_3^-$.[42]

SID theory provides a clearer understanding of the mechanism for hyperchloremic acidosis, in that intravenous administration of large volumes of a crystalloid solution, such as 0.9% NaCl or sodium gluconate, alters 2 of the 3 independent determinants of plasma pH, namely SID and A_{tot}.[23,40,41,43,44] The effect on A_{tot} is a direct and predictable effect of the volume infused; the greater the volume administered, the larger the decrease in A_{tot}. Because a decrease in A_{tot} causes a nonvolatile buffer ion alkalosis, the effect of volume infusion on A_{tot} does not provide an explanation for dilutional acidosis.[40,41] Instead, dilutional acidosis is primarily due to the effect of infusion on plasma SID; the net effect on plasma SID (and, therefore, pH) depends on both the volume infused and the SID of the infused crystalloid solution.[40,41,43–45]

The effect of intravenous crystalloid solution formulation on blood pH is best understood by plotting blood pH against the volume infused for solutions of differing SID (**Fig. 4**). Using the simplified strong ion equation[11] and experimentally determined values for A_{tot} (0.224 × [total protein in g/L]) and K_a (0.8 × 10^{-7}) of human plasma,[46] whereas assuming normal values for blood pH (7.40), Pco_2 (40 mm Hg), pK_1' (6.105), S (0.0307 [mmol/L]/mm Hg), total protein concentration (72 g/L), and SID (36 mEq/L),[17,46] the effect of infusing 4 solutions can be calculated: 0.9% NaCl solution (SID = 0 mEq/L); 5% dextrose (SID = 0 mEq/L); lactated Ringer solution (theoretic maximum SID = 28 mEq/L); and 1.3% NaHCO3 (SID = 155 mEq/L).

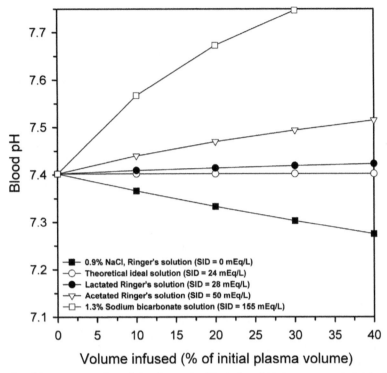

Fig. 4. Graphic representation of the theoretic effect of rapid intravenous administration of 4 crystalloid solutions on venous blood pH in humans. SID, the difference between the charge of strong cations and anions in plasma. (*Adapted from* Constable PD. In response: letters to the editor. Anesth Analg 2004;98:271–2.)

The theoretic maximum SID represents the final SID after complete metabolism of metabolizable strong anions, such as L-lactate and D-lactate in lactated Ringer (which is a racemic mixture of L-lactate and D-lactate, with D-lactate metabolism much slower than that of L-lactate). **Fig. 4** tells a clear and compelling story, 0.9% NaCl, and 5% dextrose solutions decrease plasma pH in a dose-dependent manner. Based on normal values for human plasma, the intravenous administration of a crystalloid solution with an effective SID less than 25 mEq/L is always acidifying, whereas the administration of a crystalloid solution with an effective SID greater than 25 mEq/L is always alkalinizing. This prediction has been experimentally verified by an in vitro study.[43]

The strong ion approach leads directly to the conclusion that the rapid intravenous administration of equal volumes of 0.9% NaCl, Ringer solution, sodium gluconate, 5% dextrose, and mannitol produce the same acidifying effect because the SID of all 5 solutions equals 0 mEq/L (see **Fig. 4**).[45] Current application of SID theory, therefore, explains why a similar decrease in pH occurs in dogs administered 0.9% NaCl, 5% dextrose, or 5% mannitol intravenously at 88 mL/kg body weight.[39] **Fig. 4** also provides an explanation as to why the rapid intravenous administration of large volumes (70 mL/kg) of 0.9% NaCl produces a metabolic acidosis in humans, whereas administration of equivalent volumes of lactated Ringer solution does not cause a detectable change in plasma pH.[47]

APPLICATION OF STRONG ION DIFFERENCE THEORY TO CALVES WITH DIARRHEA

The simplified strong ion equation, therefore provides a consilient scientific theory that unifies a variety of observations.[48] Application of strong ion theory provides "a comprehensive evaluation of acid-base status, the possible causes of acid-base disorders in animals, and thus a better way for treatment by calculating SID and A_{tot} values of the therapeutic fluids."[11–14,28–30,40,44,49,50] Moreover, the simplified strong ion equation has greater explanatory power than the Henderson-Hasselbalch equation because it accounts for previously unexplained phenomena. The SID approach has its critics, however, with some investigators concluding that "the Stewart approach is absurd and anachronistic" and that "the terminology is misleading, confusing anions and cations with acids and bases."[51] Other investigators have raised the question, "is the Stewart formulation a stately horse without legs?" and concluded that the strong ion approach does not provide any diagnostic advantage over the Henderson-Hasselbalch equation.[7] The same critics then invoke Occam's razor that entities should not be multiplied unnecessarily (if 2 approaches produce the same solution, then the simpler approach should be used, which is the 4-Henderson-Hasselbalch equation).

There is no need to use Stewart's equation or Constable's simplified strong ion equation instead of the simpler Henderson-Hasselbalch equation in descriptive experimental studies when the plasma protein concentration is approximately normal. This is because all 3 (pH, P_{CO2}, and [HCO_3^-]) of the 3 unknowns in the Henderson-Hasselbalch equation can be measured accurately and easily in plasma, whereas only 2 (pH and P_{CO2}) of the 4 unknowns in the simplified strong ion approach (pH, P_{CO2}, SID, and A_{tot}) can be measured accurately and easily in plasma. The simplified strong ion equation can, however, provide a valuable insight into the mechanism of an acid-base abnormality that is different from that obtained from the Henderson-Hasselbalch equation. It is, therefore, important to highlight the findings of a 2005 study in 231 sick calves (most with diarrhea) that identified important limitations in using the Henderson-Hasselbalch equation to evaluate acid-base abnormalities.[29] It had been assumed for many years that the decrease in plasma $cHCO_3^-$ in calves with diarrhea was due to excessive bicarbonate loss in the feces or consumption of bicarbonate while buffering endogenously produced acids, such as D-lactic acid or L-lactic acid. Application of the Henderson-Hasselbalch equation indicated that acidemia in diarrheic and sick calves was primarily due to a decrease in plasma $cHCO_3^-$.[29] A cursory examination, however, of the spider plot relating plasma pH to changes in plasma $cHCO_3^-$ indicates that the change in plasma $cHCO_3^-$ explained most but not all of the change in plasma pH. This is most easily appreciated by the lack of clustering of individual data points along the calculated plasma pH- $cHCO_3^-$ relationship (see **Fig. 2**). Application of the Henderson-Hasselbalch equation failed to identify hyponatremia accompanied by normochloremia or mild hyperchloremia as an important cause of acidemia in diarrheic calves and ignored the effect of hyper D-lactatemia, dehydration, and increased plasma protein concentration on acid-base balance. Moreover, the R^2 value for the Henderson-Hasselbalch regression equation was 0.03 to 0.07 lower for 4 data sets than that for the strong ion approach, indicating that the Henderson-Hasselbalch equation had less explanatory power than the strong ion approach. In comparison, application of the simplified strong ion equation to the calves provided a new and revolutionary insight into the mechanism for the acidemia. Specifically, acidemia was primarily due to decreased SID secondary to hyponatremia and increased plasma concentrations of L-lactate, D-lactate, and uremic anions (see **Figs. 1** and **3**), which all contribute to decreasing plasma SID from its normal value of 42 mEq/L. The increase in plasma protein concentration also contributed to the acidemia but to a smaller extent than SID, with the increase in plasma protein concentration resulting from the loss of free water and dehydration. SID theory, therefore, indicated that the optimal treatment of diarrheic calves with acidemia is intravenous sodium bicarbonate, which has an effective SID of 155 mEq/L and is, therefore, strongly alkalinizing. SID theory indicates that it is the sodium in sodium bicarbonate and, therefore, the SID or the intravenous fluid that is important in correcting the acid-base disturbance. In contrast, application of the Henderson-Hasselbalch equation to diarrheic calves indicates that acidemia is primarily due to decreased plasma $cHCO_3^-$ and that it is the bicarbonate in sodium bicarbonate that is important. This example demonstrates that the same recommended treatment can result from using 2 completely different approaches to analyzing acid-base balance.

Increased understanding of the pathophysiology of an acid-base disorder obviously leads to a more targeted treatment of acid-base and electrolyte disorders. In cattle, strong ion theory has clearly identified the importance of administering high SID fluids to acidemic calves[29] and that calculating the SID of oral rehydration solutions is helpful in identifying optimal solution formulation.[52-55] This example is one of many that indicate, contrary to Kurtz and colleagues'[7] conclusion, that SID theory can provide a diagnostic advantage over the Henderson-Hasselbalch equation.

COLLECTION OF BLOOD SAMPLES TO EVALUATE ACID-BASE STATUS

If the primary clinical interest is evaluation of the metabolic component of an acid-base disturbance, then a jugular venous blood sample should be anaerobically obtained in a 3-mL polypropylene syringe that has been previously coated internally with sodium heparin (by drawing sodium heparin into the syringe barrel and then expelling all heparin from the syringe into the barrel before blood collection). After blood collection, the air bubbles should be removed from the blood in the syringe by holding the syringe vertically and vigorously tapping the barrel of the syringe to cause any bubbles to coalesce and move vertically. Some blood (with the bubbles) should then be expelled to remove all air bubbles. The end of the needle is then corked to minimize the loss of CO_2 and addition of O_2 to the blood sample. The polypropylene syringe should then be stored at room temperature and analyzed within 30 minutes of collection because this causes the smallest changes in Po_2 and pH. The polypropylene syringe should not be placed in iced water ($0°C$) until analyzed because this facilitates oxygen diffusion across the barrel of the polypropylene syringe, thereby increasing the measured Po_2 value.[56] If an accurate Po_2 value is of minimal interest and blood pH is of greater concern, then blood should be stored in iced water ($0°C$) to minimize time-related changes in pH and Pco_2 due to cellular metabolism, particularly in blood samples with high white blood cell concentrations.[56] Blood pH, however, usually does not change during 30 minutes of storage at room temperature.

If the primary interest is evaluation of the respiratory system, an arterial blood sample (auricular artery in all aged cattle; median artery or saphenous artery in calves in lateral recumbency) should be obtained, handled, and stored in the same manner as for venous blood samples.

Partially evacuated tubes containing lyophilized lithium heparin have been used to collect jugular venous blood samples for blood gas and acid-base analysis in cattle.[57] A 2009 Clinical and Laboratory Standards Institute document on approved guidelines for blood gas and pH analysis does not recommend the use of partially evacuated tubes for sample collection.[19] This is because blood collected into partially evacuated tubes undergoes an immediate, sustained, and marked increase in P_{O_2} and an immediate, transient, and small decrease in P_{CO_2}. The increase in P_{O_2} is exacerbated when partially evacuated tubes are stored in iced water instead of room temperature.[58]

MEASUREMENT OF TOTAL CO₂

An extremely useful and underused screening test for acid-base status in cattle without evidence of respiratory disease is the total CO_2 concentration ($ctCO_2$) in venous plasma or serum.[13] $ctCO_2$ is defined as the amount of total carbon dioxide in plasma that can be liberated with a strong acid and can be measured by a chemical analyzer or calculated from the results of routine blood gas analysis as $ctCO_2 = cHCO_3^- +$ dissolved CO_2.[19] A decrease in $ctCO_2$ indicates a metabolic acidosis, whereas an increase in $ctCO_2$ indicates metabolic alkalosis (see **Fig. 1**).

Preanalytical errors in the measurement of $ctCO_2$ can result in an incorrect interpretation of acid-base status. Glass or plastic evacuated tubes are commonly used in veterinary medicine to collect blood samples for plasma or serum biochemical analysis. Underfilling partially evacuated tubes results in a lower measured value for $ctCO_2$ than when tubes are fully filled because CO_2 is released into the air space above the blood.[59,60] The loss of CO_2 results in a decrease in P_{CO_2} in plasma or serum after sample collection and thereby decreases plasma or serum $ctCO_2$. This decrease in P_{CO_2} and plasma or serum $ctCO_2$ is related to the ratio of blood sample volume to air volume. An unrecognized but important issue is that completely filled evacuated blood collection tubes of various sizes differ in their air volume–to–blood volume ratio and consequently the measured value for $ctCO_2$.

The air volume–to–blood volume ratio is significantly higher and, consequently, $ctCO_2$ significantly lower when blood is collected into 2-mL glass evacuated tubes and 2- or 3-mL plastic evacuated tubes than when 4-, 6-, or 10-mL plastic or glass evacuated tubes are used.[61] Consequently, blood samples should always be collected into partially evacuated tubes of 4 mL or greater size with a small air volume–to–blood volume ratio, and the tube filled as much as possible, whenever an accurate estimate of plasma or serum $ctCO_2$ is required.

QUANTIFYING THE UNMEASURED ANION CONCENTRATION

It is clinically helpful to identify the presence of unmeasured anions and quantify the unmeasured anion concentration in plasma. Unmeasured anions that are not routinely measured include L-lactate, D-lactate, β-OH butyrate, and acetoacetate as well as sulfate and anions associated with uremia. The 2 methods available to quantify the unmeasured anion concentration ([UA]) in serum or plasma are the AG and the strong ion gap (SIG) (see **Box 1**).

Anion Gap

The AG concept was derived from the concept of electroneutrality, where AG represents the difference between the [UA] and concentration of unmeasured cations ([UC]) in serum.[5,6,62,63] This is expressed by the following general equation:

$$[Na^+] + [K^+] + [UC] = [Cl^-] + [HCO_3^-] + [UA] \qquad (10)$$

Serum potassium concentration should always be included in the AG calculation in cattle because the serum potassium concentration can vary markedly. Equation (10) can be rearranged to provide

$$AG = [UA] - [UC] = ([Na^+] + [K^+]) - ([Cl^-] + [HCO_3^-]) \qquad (11)$$

This equation indicates that a change in [UA] or [UC] causes a change in the AG. An increased AG, therefore, reflects an increase in UA (likely) or a decrease in UC, which is very unlikely because quantitatively important decreases in the plasma concentration of calcium and magnesium are not compatible with life.

Normally, approximately two-thirds of the AG originates from the net negative charge of serum proteins (predominantly albumin). Because the AG is primarily dependent on the net anionic charge on serum proteins, it does not provide an accurate method for quantifying the unmeasured strong ion charge in animals with abnormal serum protein concentrations. When total protein concentrations are approximately normal, however, the AG does provide a clinically useful estimate for the concentration of unmeasured strong anions, such as L-lactate or D-lactate.

Strong Ion Gap

A useful clinical application of SID theory is calculation of the SIG instead of the AG. The SIG attributes a value to the net anionic charge on serum proteins and, therefore, provides a more accurate method for quantifying the unmeasured strong ion charge in animals with abnormal serum protein concentrations than does calculating the AG.

The SIG provides an estimate for the difference between the net strong ion charge of plasma nonvolatile buffers (albumin, globulin, and phosphate), unmeasured strong anion concentration (L-lactate, D-lactate, nonesterified fatty acids, ketoacids, pH-independent phosphate charge, sulfate, and other strong anions), and unmeasured strong cation concentrations (calcium and magnesium). The following equations can be used in cattle to calculate SIG (in mEq/L)[29]:

$$SIG = [\text{total protein}] \times (0.343/\{1 + 10^{7.08 - \text{pH}}\}) - AG \tag{12}$$

$$SIG = [\text{albumin}] \times (0.622/\{1 + 10^{7.08 - \text{pH}}\}) - AG \tag{13}$$

where [total protein] and [albumin] are in g/L and the AG (in mEq/L) = $([Na^+] + [K^+]) - ([Cl^-] + [HCO_3^-])$. Calculation from total protein concentration is preferred because both total protein and albumin are measured to 1 decimal place, with total protein concentration approximately twice the value of albumin concentration. As a result, SIG is approximately twice as sensitive to change when calculated from the total protein concentration than when calculated from the albumin concentration. An SIG greater than 0 mEq/L indicates an increase in unidentified strong cations (a rare event), whereas an SIG less than 0 mEq/L indicates an increase in unidentified strong anions, such as D-lactate, L-lactate, or uremic anions.

URINE PH AND ACID-BASE BALANCE

The most accurate insight into acid-base homeostasis in healthy cattle is obtained by measuring urine net acid excretion (NAE) or net base excretion (NBE), which is the negative value of NAE, such that NBE = −NAE. Urinary NAE has traditionally been calculated as

$$NAE = TA + [NH_4^+] - cHCO_3^- \tag{14}$$

where TA is titratable acidity and $[NH_4^+]$ is the concentration of the ammonium ion in urine. Constable and colleagues[64] recently applied SID theory to urine; this application demonstrated that the value for NAE approximated that of urine SID, which is the difference between the charge of strong cations (sodium, potassium, calcium, and magnesium) and strong anions (chloride, L-lactate, D-lactate, sulfate, ketoacids, and so forth) in urine. Additional algebraic rearrangement of the urine SID equation indicated that urine pH was related in a nonlinear manner to NBE, such that

$$pH = 6.12 + \log_{10}(NBE + [NH_4^+] + 2.5) \tag{15}$$

This equation is equivalent to the following equation:

$$pH = 6.12 + \log_{10}([K^+] + [Na^+] + [Mg^{2+}] + [Ca^{2+}] + [NH_4^+] - [Cl^-] - [SO_4^{2-}]) \tag{16}$$

with all concentrations in mEq/L.

Equations (15) and (16) were validated using a large data set from healthy cattle.[64] The validation indicated that urine pH provided an accurate assessment of systemic acid-base homeostasis in healthy cattle, but only when urine pH was greater than 6.3. Urine pH has also been associated with urine SID in neonatal calves infused with ammonium chloride.[65] Urine pH should not be used to predict systemic acid-base status in sick adult cattle because serum electrolyte abnormalities, such as hypokalemia and hypochloremia, are likely to be present with resultant changes in urine potassium and chloride concentration, and changes in these values directly alter urine pH.

SUMMARY

Clinicians who eschew SID theory but enthusiastically embrace the Henderson-Hasselbalch equation when diagnosing and treating acid-base imbalances need to recognize that they are using the simplified strong ion equation. If serum total protein, albumin, and phosphate concentrations are approximately normal, then acid-base status in cattle should be evaluated using blood pH, P_{CO_2}, and BE concentration. This is the traditional Henderson-Hasselbalch approach, with BE strongly preferred to $cHCO_3^-$ as a measure of the metabolic component of acid-base balance. The presence of unidentified anions should be investigated by calculating the AG (see **Box 1**). If serum albumin, globulin, or phosphate concentrations are abnormal, then acid-base status should be evaluated using blood pH, P_{CO_2}, measured SID, and A_{tot}. This is the simplified strong ion approach. The presence of unidentified strong ions should be investigated by calculating the SIG (see **Box 1**). Three examples of the recommended approach for evaluating acid-base balance in sick neonatal and adult ruminants are provided in Appendix 1.

REFERENCES

1. Hasselbalch KA. Die Berechnung der Wasserstoffzahl des blutes auf der freien und gebundenen Kohlensaure desselben, und die Sauerstoffbindung des Blutes als Funktion der Wasserstoffzahl. Biochem Z 1916;78:112–44.
2. Henderson LJ. The theory of neutrality regulation in the animal organism. Am J Physiol 1908;21:427–48.
3. Astrup P. A simple electrometric technique for the determination of carbon dioxide tension in blood and plasma, total content of carbon dioxide in plasma, and bicarbonate content in separated plasma at a fixed carbon dioxide tension (40 mm Hg). Scand J Clin Lab Invest 1956;8:33–43.
4. Astrup P, Jorgensen K, Siggaard-Andersen O, et al. The acid-base metabolism. A new approach. Lancet 1960;1:1035–7.
5. Oh MS, Carroll HJ. Current concepts. The anion gap. N Engl J Med 1977;297: 814–7.

6. Gabow PA. Disorders associated with an altered anion gap. Kidney Int 1985;27: 472–83.
7. Kurtz I, Kraut J, Ornekian V, et al. Acid-base analysis: a critique of the Stewart and bicarbonate-centered approaches. Am J Physiol Renal Physiol 2008; 294(5):F1009–31.
8. Stewart PA. Independent and dependent variables of acid-base control. Respir Physiol 1978;33:9–26.
9. Stewart PA. Strong ions, plus carbon dioxide, plus weak acid, isolated blood plasma and isolated intracellular fluid. In: How to understand acid-base. New York: Elsevier; 1981. p. 110–44 Chapter 7.
10. Stewart PA. Modern quantitative acid-base chemistry. Can J Physiol Pharmacol 1983;61:1444–61.
11. Constable PD. A simplified strong ion model for acid-base equilibria: application to horse plasma. J Appl Physiol 1997;83:297–311.
12. Constable PD. Clinical assessment of acid-base status: Strong ion difference theory. Fluid and electrolyte therapy. Vet Clin North Am Food Anim Pract 1999;15:447–71.
13. Constable PD. Clinical assessment of acid-base status: comparison of the Henderson-Hasselbalch and strong ion approaches. Vet Clin Pathol 2000;29:115–28.
14. Constable PD. Strong ion difference theory: a revolutionary approach to the diagnosis and treatment of acid-base abnormalities in cattle. Hungar Vet J 2008;130(Suppl 1, Keynote Lectures):28–33.
15. Baquero-Parrado JR. Consideraciones clínicas y regulación del equilibrio ácido-base en ganado bovino. Revista UDCA Actualidad & Divulgación Científica 2008;11(2):85–100.
16. Constable PD. Chapter 111. Clinical acid-base chemistry. In: Ronco C, Bellomo R, John A Kellum, editors. Critical care nephrology. 2nd edition. Philadelphia: W.B. Saunders Company; 2009. p. 581–6.
17. Austin WH, Lacombe E, Rand PW, et al. Solubility of carbon dioxide in serum from 15 to 38 C. J Appl Physiol 1963;18:301–4.
18. Rispens P, Dellebarre CW, Eleveld D, et al. The apparent first dissociation constant of carbonic acid in plasma between 16 and 42.5°. Clin Chim Acta 1968;22: 627–37.
19. Clinical and Laboratory Standards Institute. Blood gas and pH analysis and related measurements; approved guidelines. CLSI document C46-A2. 2nd edition. Wayne (PA): Clinical and Laboratory Standards Institute; 2009.
20. Tibi L, Bhattacharya SS, Flear CT. Variability in pK_1' of human plasma. Clin Chim Acta 1982;121:15–31.
21. Rosan RC, Enlander D, Ellis J. Unpredictable error in calculated bicarbonate homeostasis during pediatric intensive care: The delusion of fixed pK_1'. Clin Chem 1983;29:69–73.
22. Wooten EW. Calculation of physiological acid-base parameters in multicompartment systems with application to human blood. J Appl Physiol 2003;95:2333–44.
23. Omron EM, Omron RM. A physicochemical model of crystalloid infusion on acid-base status. J Intensive Care Med 2010;25:271–80.
24. van Slyke DD. Studies of acidosis. XVII. The normal and abnormal variations in the acid-base balance of the blood. J Biol Chem 1921;48:153–76.
25. Kofstad J. Base excess: a historical review – has the calculation of base excess been more standardized the last 20 years? Clin Chim Acta 2001;307:193–5.
26. Mentel A, Bach F, Schuler J, et al. Assessing errors in the determination of base excess. Anesth Analg 2002;94:1141–8.

27. Lightman A, Gingerich O. When do anomalies begin? Science 1991;255: 690–5.
28. Constable PD. Total weak acid concentration and effective dissociation constant of nonvolatile buffers in human plasma. J Appl Physiol 2001;91:1364–71.
29. Constable PD, Staempfli HR, Navetat H, et al. Use of a quantitative strong ion approach to determine the mechanism for acid-base abnormalities in sick calves with or without diarrhea. J Vet Intern Med 2005;19:581–9.
30. Constable PD. Calculation of variables describing plasma nonvolatile weak acids for use in the strong ion approach to acid-base balance in cattle. Am J Vet Res 2002;63:482–90.
31. van Slyke DD. Studies of gas and electrolyte equilibria in blood. XIV. The amounts of alkali bound by serum albumin and globulin. J Biol Chem 1928; 79:769–80.
32. McAuliffe JJ, Lind LJ, Leith DE, et al. Hypoproteinemic alkalosis. Am J Med 1986;81:86–90.
33. Rossing TH, Maffeo N, Fencl V. Acid-base effects of altering plasma protein concentration in human blood in vitro. J Appl Physiol 1986;61:2260–5.
34. Figge J, Mydosh T, Fencl V. Serum protein and acid-base equilibria: a follow-up. J Lab Clin Med 1992;120:713–9.
35. Lean IJ, DeGaris PJ, McNeil DM, et al. Hypocalcemia in dairy cows: Meta-analysis and dietary cation anion difference theory revisited. J Dairy Sci 2006; 89:669–84.
36. Gelfert CC, Loeffler LM, Fromer S, et al. Comparison of the impact of different anionic salts on the acid-base status and calcium metabolism in non-lactating, non-pregnant dairy cows. Vet J 2010;185:305–9.
37. Shires GT, Holman J. Dilutional acidosis. Ann Intern Med 1948;28:557–9.
38. Rehm M, Finsterer U. Treating intraoperative hyperchloremic acidosis with sodium bicarbonate or Tris-Hydroxymethyl Aminomethane; a randomized prospective study. Anesth Analg 2003;96:1201–8.
39. Asano S, Kato E, Yamauchi M, et al. The mechanism of acidosis caused by infusion of saline solution. Lancet 1966;1:1245–6.
40. Constable PD. In response: letters to the editor. Anesth Analg 2004;98:271–2.
41. Constable PD. Iatrogenic hyperchloremic acidosis due to large volume fluid administration. Int J Intens Care 2005;12(3):111.
42. Levetown M. Saline-induced hyperchloremic metabolic acidosis. Crit Care Med 2002;30:259–61.
43. Morgan TJ, Venkatesh B, Hall J. Crystalloid strong ion difference determines metabolic acid-base change during in vitro hemodilution. Crit Care Med 2002; 30:157–60.
44. Constable PD. Hyperchloremic acidosis: the classic example of strong ion acidosis. Anesth Analg 2003;96(4):919–22.
45. Müller KR, Gentile A, Klee W, et al. Importance of the effective strong ion difference of an intravenous solution in the treatment of diarrheic calves with naturally-acquired acidemia and strong ion (metabolic) acidosis. J Vet Intern Med 2012;26(3):674–83.
46. Staempfli HR, Constable PD. Experimental determination of net protein charge and A_{tot} and K_a of nonvolatile buffers in human plasma. J Appl Physiol 2003;95: 620–30.
47. Scheingraber S, Rehm M, Sehmisch C, et al. Rapid saline infusion produces hyperchloremic acidosis in patients undergoing gynecologic surgery. Anesthesiology 1999;90:1243–54.

48. Ruse M. Falsifiability, consilience, and systematics. Syst Zool 1979;29:530–6.
49. Elkhair NM, Siegling-Vlitakis C, Radtke E, et al. Age-dependent response of the acid-base parameters (Henderson-Hasselbalch, Stewart) in healthy calves with experimentally induced metabolic acidosis. Berl Munch Tierarztl Wochenschr 2009;122:63–9.
50. Hartmann H, Bachmann L. Einfluss der elektrolyte in oralen rehydratationslösungen auf das labmagenmileau und den systemischen säuren-basen-staus mit hinweisen zur behandlung der diarrhoe bei kalbern. Klauentierpraxis 2007;15:117–22.
51. Siggaard-Andersen O, Fogh-Andersen N. Base excess or buffer base (strong ion difference) as measure of a non-respiratory acid-base disturbance. Acta Anaesthesiol Scand 1995;39(Suppl 107):123–8.
52. Bachmann L, Berchtold J, Siegling-Vlitakis C, et al. Stewart variables of the acid-base status in calves. Age related behavior and influence of spontaneously occurring diarrhea. Tierarztl Praxis 2009;37:365–74.
53. Bachmann L, Homeier T, Arlt S, et al. Influence of different oral rehydration solutions on abomasal conditions and the acid-base status of suckling calves. J Dairy Sci 2009;92:1649–59.
54. Staempfli H, Oliver O, Pringle JK. Clinical evaluation of an oral electrolyte solution formulated based on strong ion difference (SID) and using propionate as the organic anion in the treatment of neonatal diarrheic calves with strong ion acidosis. Open J Vet Med 2012;2:34–9.
55. Constable PD, Thomas E, Boisrame B. Comparison of two oral electrolyte solutions for the treatment of dehydrated calves with experimentally-induced diarrhoea. Vet J 2001;162(2):129–41.
56. Kennedy SA, Constable PD, Sen I, et al. Effects of syringe type and storage conditions on results of equine blood gas and acid-base analysis. Am J Vet Res 2012;73(7):979–87.
57. Donovan DC, Hippen AR, Hurley DJ, et al. The role of acidogenic diets and β-hydroxybutyrate on lymphocyte proliferation and serum antibody response against bovine respiratory viruses in Holstein steers. J Anim Sci 2003;81:3088–94.
58. Noel PG, Couetil L, Constable PD. Effects of collecting blood into plastic heparinized Vacutainer tubes and storage conditions on blood gas analysis values in horses. Equine Vet J 2010;42(Suppl 38):91–7.
59. Herr RD, Swanson T. Serum bicarbonate declines with sample size in Vacutainer tubes. Am J Clin Pathol 1992;97:213–6.
60. James KM, Polzin DJ, Osborne CA, et al. Effects of sample handling on total carbon dioxide concentrations in canine and feline serum and blood. Am J Vet Res 1997;58:343–7.
61. Tinkler SH, Couëtil LL, Kennedy SA, et al. Effect of the size of evacuated blood collection tubes on total carbon dioxide concentration in equine plasma. J Am Vet Med Assoc 2012;241(7):922–6.
62. Constable PD, Streeter RK, Koenig GR, et al. Determinants and utility of the anion gap in predicting hyperlactatemia in cattle. J Vet Intern Med 1997;11:71–9.
63. Constable PD, Hinchcliff KW, Muir WW. Comparison of anion gap and strong ion gap as predictors of unmeasured strong ion concentration in plasma and serum from horses. Am J Vet Res 1998;59:881–7.
64. Constable PD, Gelfert CC, Fürll M, et al. Application of strong ion difference theory to urine and the relationship between urine pH and net acid excretion in cattle. Am J Vet Res 2009;70:915–25.
65. Elkhair NM, Hartmann H. Studies on acid-base status in calves with ammonium chloride induced metabolic acidosis. Global Vet 2012;9:388–95.

APPENDIX 1

Three examples of the recommended approach for evaluating acid-base balance in sick neonatal and adult ruminants are discussed.

Case 1. A 4-year-old lactating Holstein-Friesian cow (668-kg body weight) was diagnosed with a left displaced abomasum based on a left-sided ping located from the 10th to the 13th ribs. The cow had been off-feed for 4 days (dry matter intake <15 kg/d = 2.2% body weight/d), was not clinically dehydrated, and had profound ketonemia (plasma β-OH butyrate concentration = 6.8 mmol/L; plasma nonesterified fatty acid concentration = 1.2 mmol/L; and plasma glucose concentration = 33 mg/dL {1.8 mmol/L}), profound ketonuria (urine acetoacetate concentration, >80 mg/dL by semiquantitative sodium nitroprusside reaction), and aciduria (urine pH = 6.0). The heart rate was 72 beats/min, the rectal temperature was 100.9°F (38.3°C), the respiratory rate was 26 breaths/min, and normal breath sounds were heard on thoracic auscultation. Ruminal hypomotility was evident (rumen contraction rate, 3/3 min). Additional laboratory results are shown in **Table 1**.

Interpretation: the absence of respiratory disease means that total CO_2 provides a good screening test for acid-base evaluation, which indicates the absence of a major metabolic abnormality. The Henderson-Hasselbalch equation can be used to evaluate acid-base balance because the plasma total protein concentration was within the reference range. Hypokalemia in an adult ruminant with normal blood pH suggests the presence of whole-body potassium depletion. The low urine pH (6.0) was suggestive of the presence of metabolic acidosis and acidemia; however, urine pH is not an accurate indicator of systemic acid-balance in diseased ruminants because of the likely concurrent presence of electrolyte abnormalities. Additional laboratory testing indicated low urinary fractional clearance of K (52% urine), consistent with the clinical

Table 1
Laboratory results in Case 1

Plasma Constituent	Value	Reference Range	Interpretation
Routine screening parameter			
Total CO_2 (mEq/L)	29.1	28–34	Normal
Henderson-Hasselbalch equation			
pH	7.36	7.38–7.46	Acidemia (mild)
P_{CO_2} (mm Hg)	50	42–52	Normal
$cHCO_3$ (mmol/L)	27.6	27–33	Normal
SBE (mEq/L)	2.4	2–8	Normal
AG (mEq/L)	20.3	14–20	Increased (mild)
Simplified strong ion model			
Na^+ (mEq/L)	137	136–148	Normal
K^+ (mEq/L)	2.9	3.4–4.8	Hypokalemia
Cl^- (mEq/L)	92	90–102	Normal
$SID_{measured}$ (mEq/L)	47.9	38–46	Mild strong ion alkalosis
Total protein (g/L)	64	60–76	Normal
A_{tot} (mmol/L)	22.0	20–26	Normal
A_{tot} (mEq/L)	14.9	14–18	Normal
SIG (mEq/L)	−5.4	−2 to +6	↑ Unidentified strong anions

impression that aciduria was most likely due to whole-body potassium depletion and, therefore, low urine potassium concentration.

Blood gas analysis indicated a mild acidemia (decreased blood pH) that could not be specifically attributed to respiratory or metabolic acidosis. The mild increase in AG suggested the presence of unmeasured anions, most likely strong anion, such as β-OH butyrate because the plasma total protein concentration was within the reference range.

The simplified strong ion approach reveals severe strong ion alkalosis, primarily due to marked hypochloremia. Calculation of the SIG, however, reveals the presence of unidentified strong ions, most likely ketoacids, such as β-OH butyrate and nonesterified fatty acids. This example highlights a potential error when using the measured SID to evaluate the presence or absence of a strong ion abnormality (which is best evaluated by calculating the SIG). The most appropriate treatment for this cow is specific treatment of ketosis, fat mobilization, and hypokalemia.

Case 2. A 9-day-old Holstein-Friesian heifer calf was examined because of profound weakness, inappetence, and marked dehydration due to diarrhea of 3 days' duration. The calf had received 3 L of first milking colostrum within 2 hours of birth. The heart rate was 144 beats/min, the rectal temperature was 35.2°C, the respiratory rate was 24 breaths/min, and normal breath sounds were heard on thoracic auscultation. The calf was estimated to be 10% dehydrated based on an eye recession into the orbit of 6 mm. Additional laboratory results are shown in **Table 2**.

Interpretation: the severe dehydration suggests that total protein concentration may be increased and that the simplified strong ion approach should be used. The high total protein concentration confirms that the simplified strong ion approach should be used.

The blood pH indicates profound acidemia, which is due to a strong anion acidosis (based on the very negative SIG) and to a lesser extent a nonvolatile buffer ion acidosis

Table 2
Laboratory results in Case 2

Plasma Constituent	Value	Normal Range	Interpretation
Routine screening parameter			
Total CO_2 (mEq/L)	10.5	24–30	Metabolic acidosis (profound)
Henderson-Hasselbalch equation			
pH	6.96	7.32–7.40	Acidemia (profound)
P_{CO_2} (mm Hg)	42	45–55	Respiratory alkalosis (mild)
$cHCO_3$ (mmol/L)	9.2	23–29	Metabolic acidosis (profound)
SBE (mEq/L)	−21.7	0–6	Metabolic acidosis (profound)
AG (mEq/L)	37.9	21–34	↑ Unidentified anions (marked)
Simplified strong ion model			
Na^+ (mEq/L)	135	137–145	Hyponatremia (mild)
K^+ (mEq/L)	7.1	4.7–5.5	Hyperkalemia (moderate)
Cl^- (mEq/L)	95	92–98	Normal
$SID_{measured}$ (mEq/L)	47.1	38–46	Strong ion alkalosis (mild)
Total protein (g/L)	79	51–59	Hyperproteinemia (marked)
A_{tot} (mmol/L)	27.1	11–19	Nonvolatile buffer ion acidosis
A_{tot} (mEq/L)	11.7	11–19	Normal net protein charge
SIG (mEq/L)	−26.2	−2 to +6	Marked ↑ unidentified strong anions

(based on the increased plasma total protein concentration). Unidentified strong ions are present, most likely L-lactate, D-lactate, and strong anions associated with uremia. Plasma L-lactate concentration was measured and determined to be 3.1 mmol/L; this suggested the presence of a large concentration of D-lactate and uremic anions in plasma. Calculation of the AG did not reveal the marked increase in the unmeasured strong anion concentration that was indicated by calculating the SIG. This is partly because the AG includes the effect of changes in net plasma protein charge, which in turn is dependent on the plasma protein concentration as well as the plasma pH.

Correction of the acid-base disturbance in this calf requires the intravenous administration of an isotonic solution with a high effective SID (such as 1.3% or 1.4% sodium bicarbonate solution) to increase the actual plasma SID, decrease the plasma protein concentration, and increase renal blood flow, glomerular filtration rate, and urine production in order for D-lactate and uremic anions to be cleared from the plasma.

Case 3. A 3-year-old Holstein-Friesian cow was diagnosed with an abomasal volvulus based on the presence of a large right-sided ping spanning the 8th rib to caudal to the 13th rib, a splashing sound on succussion of the right abdominal quadrant, and a large viscus in the cranial right quadrant detected by palpation per rectum. The cow has had decreased appetite and milk production for 1 day, was clinically dehydrated, and was not ketonemic (plasma β-OH butyrate concentration = 0.8 mmol/L). The heart rate was 88 beats/min, the rectal temperature was 100.4°F (38.0°C), respiratory rate was 32 breaths/min, and normal breath sounds were heard on thoracic auscultation. Ruminal hypomotility was evident (rumen contraction rate, 1 per 2 minutes). The plasma L-lactate concentration was 2.6 mmol/L. Additional laboratory results are shown in **Table 3**.

Interpretation: the absence of respiratory disease means that total CO_2 provides a good screening test for acid-base evaluation, which indicates the presence of marked

Table 3
Laboratory results in Case 3

Plasma Constituent	Value	Normal Range	Interpretation
Routine screening parameter			
Total CO_2 (mEq/L)	49.8	28–34	Metabolic acidosis
Henderson-Hasselbalch equation			
pH	7.46	7.38–7.46	Normal
P_{CO_2} (mm Hg)	66	42–52	Respiratory acidosis (moderate)
$cHCO_3$ (mmol/L)	47.8	27–33	Metabolic alkalosis (profound)
BE (mEq/L)	23.8	2–8	Metabolic alkalosis (profound)
AG (mEq/L)	28.0	14–20	Increased unidentified anions
Simplified strong ion model			
Na^+ (mEq/L)	143	136–148	Normal
K^+ (mEq/L)	2.8	3.4–4.8	Hypokalemia
Cl^- (mEq/L)	70	90–102	Hypochloremia (marked)
$SID_{measured}$ (mEq/L)	75.8	38–46	Strong ion alkalosis (profound)
Total protein (g/L)	97	60–76	Hyperproteinemia (marked)
A_{tot} (mmol/L)	33.3	20–26	Nonvolatile buffer ion acidosis
A_{tot} (mEq/L)	23.5	14–18	Increased net protein charge
SIG (mEq/L)	−4.5	−2 to +6	↑ Unidentified strong anions

metabolic alkalosis. Because of the presence of abomasal volvulus, a marked hypchloremic, hypokalemic, metabolic alkalosis is assumed. The high total protein concentration indicates that the simplified strong ion approach should be used.

The presence of respiratory acidosis (increased P_{CO_2}) and nonvolatile buffer ion acidosis (increased A_{tot}) in the presence of a blood pH on the high end of the reference range suggests the presence of a marked strong ion acidosis. This is confirmed by the extremely high value for $SID_{measured}$ (75.8 mEq/L) in the absence of a large concentration of unmeasured strong anions (the increased strong gap of −4.5 mEq/L could be accounted for primarily by the small increase in plasma L-lactate concentration).

Correction of the acid-base disturbance in this cow requires decreasing the plasma SID by increasing the serum chloride concentration and providing free water to decrease the plasma protein concentration. The most appropriate treatment is therefore surgical correction of the abomasal volvulus (which permits intestinal absorption of sequestered chloride, potassium, and water) in conjunction with an isotonic intravenous solution such as Ringer solution (which has the highest chloride concentration) or 0.9% NaCl solution with supplemental oral KCl (up to 240 g over first 24 hours).

D-Lactic Acidosis in Neonatal Ruminants

Ingrid Lorenz, Dr med vet, Dr med vet habil[a],*, Arcangelo Gentile, Dr med vet[b]

KEYWORDS

- D-lactic acidosis • Ruminants • Neonates • Calf diarrhea • Ruminal drinking

KEY POINTS

- D-Lactic metabolic acidosis in neonatal ruminants is caused by absorption of D-lactic acid abnormally produced and accumulated in the rumen or the intestines as a result of fermentation of easily fermentable carbohydrates.
- D-Lactic metabolic acidosis can develop after ruminal drinking as a result of dysfunction of the esophageal groove reflex.
- D-Lactic metabolic acidosis is a common complication of neonatal calf diarrhea, and it is responsible for most of the clinical signs, such as depression and ataxia.
- Syndromes of D-lactic acidosis without dehydration and with no, or minimal, diarrhea occur in calves, goat kids, and lambs. The cause is so far unknown.
- Serum D-lactate concentrations regularly decrease after complete correction of metabolic acidosis, and when necessary, dehydration, in affected animals.

Videos of calves with metabolic acidosis/D-Lactatemia accompany this article at http://www.vetfood.theclinics.com/

Until the 1980s, D-lactic metabolic acidosis was known to occur only in adult ruminants caused by acute ruminal acidosis as a result of carbohydrate overload.[1] Metabolic acidosis in calves with neonatal diarrhea was believed to be mainly caused by the loss of bicarbonate via the intestines or the formation of L-lactate during anaerobic glycolysis after tissue hypoperfusion in dehydrated calves. Because D-lactate was not considered to be of interest in human or veterinary medicine, routine diagnostic methods targeted the detection of L-lactate only. The development of stereospecific assays for the measurement of D-lactate[2,3] facilitated research in the area, so that our knowledge on the subject has multiplied over the last decade. This article summarizes the available information on D-lactic metabolic acidosis in neonatal ruminants.

The authors have nothing to disclose.
[a] UCD School of Veterinary Medicine, University College Dublin, Belfield, Dublin 4, Ireland;
[b] Department of Veterinary Medical Sciences, University of Bologna, 50, 40064 Ozzano Emilia, Bologna, Italy
* Corresponding author.
E-mail address: ingrid.lorenz@ucd.ie

METABOLISM OF D-LACTATE

In mammals, D-lactatemia is mainly of gastrointestinal origin. The small quantity of D-lactate that is formed in eukaryotic cells through the methylglyoxal pathway seems to be negligible.[4]

Corresponding to the experience with acute ruminal acidosis in veterinary medicine,[1] when in 1979, D-lactic acidosis was first described in humans in a patient affected by short bowel syndrome who presented with neurologic manifestations and severe metabolic acidosis,[5] the accumulation of D-lactate was attributed to the absorption of D-lactate abnormally fermented in the colon and not adequately removed because of the lack of specific metabolic pathways. At that time, it was believed that mammals metabolize D-lactate slowly, because of the lack of the specific enzyme D-lactate dehydrogenase. D-α-hydroxy acid dehydrogenase, an intramitochondrial flavoprotein enzyme, was considered the only nonspecific enzyme that initiates the metabolism of D-lactate.[6,7]

In subsequent decades, evidence was provided by different studies that mammals are able to metabolize D-lactate more efficiently than originally suggested.

Oh and colleagues[8] showed that normal humans were able to metabolize D-lactate at a rate of 1.52 mmol/kg/h at a serum level of 5.2 mmol/L, when DL-lactate was infused intravenously (IV) at a rate of 1.92 mmol/kg/h for each stereoisomer. In this study, 75% to 90% of infused D-lactate was metabolized, depending on the infusion rate. The renal threshold of D-lactate is lower than that of L-lactate, and both stereoisomers compete with each other for renal tubular reabsorption, so that a considerable proportion of D-lactate escaped through the kidneys in this experiment. Giesecke and colleagues[9] found only an average 1.2% to 2.2% of oral DL-lactic acid loads from 50 to 200 mg/kg body weight (BW) in the urine. de Vrese and colleagues[10] established a half-life of 21 minutes for D-lactate in the blood of healthy humans given an oral load of 6.4 mmol/kg BW. When a higher dose of 12.8 mmol/kg BW was used, half-life increased to 40 minutes. Less than 2% of D-lactate was excreted via the kidneys in this study.

As further evidence that D-lactate is readily metabolized by mammals, Flick and Konieczny[11] identified D-lactate dehydrogenases in mammalian tissues, capable of converting D-lactate into pyruvate, and providing therefore a glycolysis bypass for pyruvate formation from dihydroxyacetone phosphate. More recently Ling and colleagues[12] have shown that D-lactate dehydrogenase activity is high in rat liver cells, whereas it is low in brain and heart tissue.

Both stereoisomers of lactic acid are produced in the gastrointestinal tract of ruminants under physiologic conditions, and considerable amounts of D-lactic and L-lactic acid can be ingested with fermented feeds. In their basic studies on lactic acidosis in cattle after engorgement with highly fermentable carbohydrates, Dunlop and Hammond[1] found concentrations of D-lactate of up to 10 mmol/L in the blood of affected animals.

After separate infusion of the sodium salts of the 2 stereoisomers, a slower decline in blood concentration followed the infusion of sodium D-lactate. Later, it was shown that the volume of distribution for D-lactate after a single IV injection of DL-lactate was 23.5% and 24% of BW in a cow and in sheep, respectively, and 31.5% in 4 goats.[13] The latter finding was most probably because the goats that were used in this experiment were younger. The half-life of D-lactate increased with increasing concentrations of D-lactate, and goats eliminated D-lactate twice as fast as sheep and the cow in this study.[14] The renal threshold concentrations of D-lactate show differences between species, but in general, they are about half as high as the values for L-lactate. In goats, a renal threshold for D-lactate of 1.9 mmol/L was found, whereas the value for sheep and cow was 4.3 mmol/L.[15]

Induction of high concentrations of D-lactate by injection of 100 mL of a 25% sodium-D-lactate solution (223.07 mmol) in healthy calves led to a higher plasma half-time of D-lactate (183 minutes) than that reported before. Nevertheless, it was shown in this study that young calves are able to eliminate considerable amounts of D-lactate from the blood. The mean value for renal clearance was lower than that given for glomerular filtration rate[16] and thus gives strong evidence of tubular reabsorption of D-lactate. The fact that total clearance and the clearance of the 2-compartment model were higher than renal clearance indicated metabolic utilization of D-lactate by the calves.[17]

ORIGIN OF D-LACTATE IN NEONATAL RUMINANTS

Regardless of the fact that D-lactate can be theoretically introduced through ingestion of fermented feed (spoiled milk or feeding of yogurt instead of milk), the origin of D-lactate in neonatal ruminants is for practical purposes caused by fermentative processes that occur in the reticuloruminal compartment or in the intestinal tract.

Production of D-Lactate in the Reticulorumen

The mechanisms of the production and absorption of D-lactate from the rumen of adult ruminants suffering from acute ruminal acidosis caused by carbohydrate overload have been known since the middle of the last century.[1] After the first reports of the clinical picture of ruminal drinking, it seemed reasonable to assume that lactic fermentation could also be the cause of ruminal acidosis in calves.

In repeated analyses of ruminal fluid of 37 ruminal drinkers, Dirr[18] found 2 different predominant types of fermentative acidification: lactic and butyric, or both in temporal sequence. However, lactic fermentation was the one found in most ruminal drinkers. On the day of hospitalization of the animal, the concentrations of these stereoisomers was 10 ± 10 mmol/L for D-lactic acid and 31 ± 13 mmol/L for L-lactic acid, respectively, in the 20 calves with lactic acid fermentation.

High concentrations of lactic acid (up to values of 60 mmol/L) in the rumen were also reached after experimental force-feeding of whole milk; however, the stereoisomers were not measured separately in this study.[19]

Force-feeding of different oral rehydration solutions led to ruminal acidosis in all cases; however, the extent of acidification and the distribution between D-lactate and L-lactate depended strongly on the composition of the administered solutions. The concentrations of total lactic acid in the ruminal fluids in this experiment reached up to 90 mmol/L, with L-lactate being the predominant stereoisomer.[20] Gentile and colleagues[21] repeated this experiment by force-feeding calves with milk replacers. The ruminal acidosis was accompanied by concentrations of total lactic acid up to around 155.8 mmol/L. The 2 lactate stereoisomers were equally represented. To complete the spectrum of substrate potentially responsible for ruminal acidosis, Gentile and colleagues[22] force-fed whole milk, which led to intraruminal concentrations of lactic acid up to 94 mmol/L, with the 2 lactate stereoisomers equally represented.

All these studies confirmed that similarly to adult cattle, both stereoisomers of lactic acid can be abundantly produced in the rumen when easily fermentable carbohydrates contained in milk, milk replacer, or oral rehydration solutions enter the reticulorumen and are fermented by the ruminal flora in calves.

Production of D-Lactate in Neonatal Calf Diarrhea

Carbohydrates that escape digestion and absorption in the small intestine because of enteritis represent a rich fermentative substrate for colonic bacteria growing in the large intestine. The subsequent acidification of the intestinal milieu favors lactic acid producers, resulting in generation of larger amounts of L-lactic and D-lactic acids.

Several studies found increased D-lactate concentration in the feces of diarrheic calves when compared with healthy controls,[23–25] which suggests the intestines as a source of D-lactate. The fact that D-lactic metabolic acidosis was shown in diarrheic calves without increase of D-lactate concentrations in the rumen[24,26,27] further strengthens this hypothesis.

In calves with neonatal diarrhea, the risk of developing D-lactic metabolic acidosis is age dependent. In a study including 121 animals,[28] calves that suffered from diarrhea within their first 6 days of life had significantly higher base excess and significantly lower D-lactate concentrations than older calves (**Figs. 1** and **2**). Koch and Kaske[29] described that calves infected with enterotoxigenic *Escherichia coli* were younger and less acidemic than calves suffering from neonatal diarrhea caused by viral or *Cryptosporidium* infections. This finding is compatible with the hypothesis that an increase in production of D-lactate in diarrheic calves results from villous atrophy in the small intestine with maldigestion and malabsorption and subsequent microbial fermentation of substrates in the large intestine.[25]

In a study investigating D-lactate concentrations throughout the gastrointestinal tract of calves that have been euthanized for various medical reasons,[30] increased D-lactate concentrations were found throughout the gastrointestinal tract in some calves. In these calves, significantly more gram-positive rods could be found in the abomasum, the distal part of the jejunum, the cecum, and the colon when D-lactate was present (>3 mmol/L), compared with cases with negligible concentrations of D-lactate at the respective locations. It can only be speculated as to whether D-lactate is produced throughout the whole intestinal tract, or only in circumscribed areas and subsequently distributed by means of intestinal motility.

Production of D-Lactate in Acidosis Without Dehydration Syndromes

It is likely that D-lactic metabolic acidosis without dehydration and no or minimal diarrhea in the different ruminant species is also caused by overproduction of D-lactate in the intestines. Goat kids with D-lactic acidosis (floppy kid disease [FKD]) had

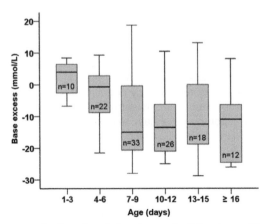

Fig. 1. Base excess concentrations in relation to age in 121 calves with neonatal diarrhea. (*From* Trefz F, Lorch A, Feist M, et al. Metabolic acidosis in neonatal calf diarrhea–clinical findings and theoretical assessment of a simple treatment protocol. J Vet Intern Med 2012;26:166; with permission.)

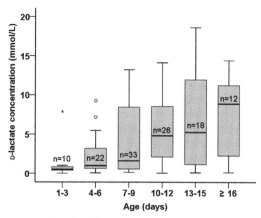

Fig. 2. D-Lactate concentrations in relation to age in 121 calves with neonatal diarrhea (○ indicates mild outliers; * indicates extreme outliers). (*From* Trefz F, Lorch A, Feist M, et al. Metabolic acidosis in neonatal calf diarrhea–clinical findings and theoretical assessment of a simple treatment protocol. J Vet Intern Med 2012;26:166; with permission.)

significantly greater colony-forming unit counts for enterococci, streptococci, staphylococci, and lactobacilli in their feces than healthy kids, which points to dysbacteria of unknown origin as the cause of the D-lactate accumulation in these animals.[31] However, the underlying pathophysiologic mechanisms leading to the suggested shift in the intestinal bacteria are not known.

CLINICAL SIGNS OF D-LACTATEMIA

Main clinical signs observed in humans with D-lactic metabolic acidosis are altered mental status, slurred speech, ataxia, disorientation, and weakness. In some cases, episodes of hostile behavior occurred.[32]

Ataxia and depression are also the most common clinical signs reported in studies investigating clinical indicators of metabolic acidosis in calves.[33–39]

However, a study on diarrheic calves with moderate to severe acidosis first suggested that D-lactate, rather than metabolic acidosis per se, was associated with impaired posture, behavior, and especially, impairment of the palpebral reflex (Video 1; available online at http://www.vetfood.theclinics.com/), whereas the sucking reflex appeared to be influenced by dehydration and metabolic acidosis.[40]

In the meantime, this hypothesis was confirmed by a series of experimental studies:

Experimentally induced severe D-lactatemia without acidosis resulted in profound changes in posture and behavior in 5 healthy calves, which could be clearly differentiated from a control group receiving 0.9% sodium chloride. All experimental calves showed impaired palpebral reflex (Video 1), with 3 calves somnolent and the remaining 2 appeared quiet and withdrawn. All calves had a staggering, drunken gait (Video 2; available online at http://www.vetfood.theclinics.com/), which was marked in 4 calves. In 4 calves, long periods of motionless or slightly wavering/tottering standing with lowered head and drooping ears were recorded (Video 3; available online at http://www. vetfood.theclinics.com/). Four calves lay down more often or for longer periods than control calves and needed help to rise. All but 1 calf assumed unphysiologic postures while standing (eg, sawhorse stance) or lying (eg, 1 foreleg extended backwards parallel to the body) for prolonged periods. No impairment of the sucking reflex could be observed in any of the calves. In this blinded study,[17] calves received an injection of 100 mL of a 25% sodium-D-lactate solution (223.07 mmol).

Induction of hyperchloremic metabolic acidosis with a mean base deficit of up to 22.4 mmol/L with an IV infusion of 4000 mL of a solution containing 400 mmol HCl in 0.9% NaCl over a period of 80 minutes in healthy calves did not cause any central nervous system signs (Video 4; available online at http://www.vetfood.theclinics.com/).[41] However, in prolonged HCl-induced metabolic acidosis, a mild depression of neurologic function could be observed.[42] In this study, acidosis was produced by infusion of either isomolar DL-lactic acid, L-lactic acid, or HCl, respectively, over a period of 6 hours. Only DL-lactic acidosis was associated with severe disturbances in neurologic functions (ie, ataxia, and depressed menace, palpebral and tactile reflexes), whereas either form of acidosis triggered depression of the sucking reflex.[42]

The fact that the impairment of the palpebral reflex (Video 1) is highly specific for D-lactic metabolic acidosis was confirmed recently by Trefz and colleagues,[43] who described a clinical picture characterized by general weakness similar to D-lactic metabolic acidosis in diarrheic calves, which is caused by hyperkalemia. The impairment or promptness of the palpebral reflex was found to be a good clinical indicator that allows a distinction to be made between these 2 disorders. Potassium and D-lactate concentrations are negatively correlated in diarrheic calves, which makes the occurrence of D-lactic acidosis and hyperkalemia simultaneously unlikely.[44]

PATHOGENESIS OF NEUROLOGIC SIGNS IN D-LACTATEMIA

Abeysekara and colleagues[42] have shown that D-lactate values in cerebrospinal fluid of calves correlated to serum concentrations after infusion of DL-lactic acid, although cerebrospinal fluid concentrations were lower and also lagged behind changes in serum concentrations.

It was hypothesized that D-lactate interfered with pyruvate metabolism because of the similarities between inherited and acquired abnormalities in pyruvate metabolism and D-lactic metabolic acidosis.[45] Studies on mitochondria from different rat tissues have recently confirmed that D-lactate is not only a poor substrate for energy production in the brain when compared with pyruvate and L-lactate but its presence also impairs the energy production from pyruvate and L-lactate.[12] These findings, together with indications that it is L-lactate, and not glucose, that is preferentially metabolized by neurons in the brain of mammals,[46,47] strengthen the hypothesis that the neurologic signs of D-lactic metabolic acidosis are caused by impairment of the energy production in the neurons.

CLINICAL SYNDROMES CAUSED BY D-LACTIC METABOLIC ACIDOSIS IN NEONATAL RUMINANTS
D-Lactic Metabolic Acidosis in Ruminal Drinkers

Fermentative intraruminal disorders (ruminal acidosis) that occur when dysfunction of the esophageal groove reflex allows milk to spill into the reticulorumen (ruminal drinking) instead of being delivered directly into the abomasum can be a starting point for D-lactic metabolic acidosis in young calves.[22,48]

Although the first descriptions of ruminal drinking were in veal calves,[49] D-lactic metabolic acidosis in ruminal drinkers has since been found[18] to occur mainly when the dysfunction of the reticular groove reflex is a complication of various primary diseases (particularly neonatal diarrhea) in artificially fed dairy calves. The early studies on reticular groove dysfunction–induced ruminal acidosis were not accompanied by the determination of serum D-lactate, but the clinical descriptions reported at that time might support that assumption. Ruminal drinking syndrome in veal calves was reported as a chronic disease characterized mainly by unthriftiness, poor appetite, retarded growth, a dull hair coat, and claylike feces.[49] On the contrary, ruminal drinking as a complication of various primary diseases in dairy calves was described as an acute process characterized by weakness, depression, prolonged recumbency, reluctance to move, inappetence, dehydration, cardiocirculatory collapse, and frequent lethal outcome.[18] This clinical picture is similar to the clinical picture that was later described as typical for D-lactic metabolic acidosis.[40]

Two forms of ruminal acidosis in calves have therefore been differentiated: an acute and a chronic form.[50] In acute ruminal acidosis, the dysfunction of the esophageal groove usually occurs secondary to diseases with systemic effects, such as neonatal diarrhea,[51] primary anorexia, and force-feeding,[52,53] or painful situations (eg, painful cough, otitis, or phlebitis of the jugular vein).[50] In chronic ruminal acidosis, the failure of the reticular groove reflex occurs in initially healthy calves and is caused by stress factors (such as prolonged transportation to assembly centers and onwards to fattening units or new groupings) or suboptimal feeding practices (eg, irregular feeding times, poor quality milk replacer, cold temperature of the milk, drinking from an open bucket).[54]

The first evidence for esophageal groove dysfunction as a severe complication of neonatal diarrhea was provided by Dirksen and Dirr in 1989.[51] In their study, 28 (11.2%) of 249 calves affected by neonatal diarrhea were confirmed as in addition suffering from ruminal acidosis. Although the clinical findings were not reported, the severity of the condition can be deduced by the fact that 11 (39.3%) of the 28 ruminal drinkers died or had to be euthanized during the hospitalization, as opposed to less than 20% in uncomplicated diarrhea.

Acute ruminal acidosis can also be induced by force-feeding of calves that are anorexic because of underlying diseases, in which case the prognosis deteriorates even further.[55,56]

A series of experiments aimed to investigate the clinical repercussions of ruminal acidosis caused by ruminal drinking indicated that the composition of the liquid entering the reticulorumen is likely to be one of the factors influencing the severity of the clinical signs.[19–22] The most distinct clinical signs (marked depression, severe dehydration, absence of sucking reflex, lack of appetite, prolonged recumbency) were observed after intraruminal administration of whole milk.[19,22] After force-feeding of milk replacer, clinical findings were limited to transitory dullness and reduced growth rate when compared with control calves,[21] and also the intraruminal administration of oral rehydration solutions provoked less severe clinical signs than that of whole milk.[20]

In a retrospective study on 293 calves younger than 4 weeks, in which ruminal acidosis (pH<6) was diagnosed on hospitalization, Gentile and colleagues[48] found a high anion gap metabolic acidosis, with the highest values in the group of calves with ruminal pH less than 5. Metabolic acidosis was not only present in animals with diarrhea or with a history of diarrhea but also in the group of calves admitted without any history of diarrhea. In this group, 46 of 91 calves (50.5%) showed metabolic acidosis, with the highest prevalence in the subgroup with ruminal pH less than 5 (39/54 = 72.2%). Because the measured L-lactate values were within the physiologic range, D-lactate was suspected as the cause of the increase of the anion gap; however, serum D-lactate concentrations were not available. A similar conclusion was drawn by Stocker and colleagues,[57] who found a high anion gap metabolic acidosis in 50 calves with chronic indigestion caused by ruminal drinking. Neither of the lactate stereoisomers was determined in this study. A mild metabolic acidosis was also observed after prolonged intraruminal administration of milk replacers.[21] Only L-lactate was measured in this study, which constantly remained within the physiologic range.

Gentile and colleagues[22] were able to provoke severe D-lactic metabolic acidosis in 8 of 9 experimental calves after intraruminal administration of whole milk. The most severe metabolic aberrations were reached after the first 10 days of the study, during which the pH of the ruminal fluid was constantly less than 4.5. At this point, mean calculated base excess was −10.0 mmol/L (±7.89), anion gap 22.5 mmol/L (±3.31), and serum D-lactate level 8.5 mmol/L (±2.1). D-Lactatemia reached peak values of 6.75 to 11.5 mmol/L in individual calves. Force-feeding was discontinued in 7 of 9 calves because of profound clinical or metabolic alterations (severe depression, estimated degree of dehydration >10%, absence of sucking reflex, lack of appetite for 2 consecutive feedings, severe metabolic acidosis with calculated actual base excess less than −15 mmol/L). Despite increased D-lactate concentrations, 2 calves developed no distinct clinical signs up to the end of the study at day 17. L-lactate constantly remained within the physiologic ranges in all calves.

It is obvious that D-lactic metabolic acidosis in calves can be caused by ruminal acidosis as a result of fermentation of carbohydrate rich solutions in the reticulorumen. However, because ruminal acidosis most often occurs as a complication of other disorders, it is in many cases difficult to distinguish the contribution of the lactate production in the rumen to the clinical and metabolic alterations in individual cases.

Metabolic Acidosis Without Dehydration Syndrome in Suckler Calves

Schelcher and colleagues[58] confirmed D-lactic acid as the cause of a syndrome of high anion gap metabolic acidosis in suckler calves with no dehydration and no or minimal diarrhea. Mean values of up to approximately 13 mmol/L were found in affected calves, with values of 1.27 ± 1.14 and 2.31 ± 1.61 mmol/L, respectively, for healthy controls in 2 consecutive years. The acidosis without dehydration syndrome was first described in 1984 by Kasari and Naylor,[33] who identified unconsciousness or depression, weakness, and ataxia as the main clinical signs. These investigators identified an increased anion gap; however, they were unable to determine the causative organic acid, because the concentrations of L-lactate, acetate, and acetoacetate were normal, and the concentration of D-lactate was not measured.

D-Lactic Metabolic Acidosis in Neonatal Calf Diarrhea

An investigation[26] into the metabolic consequences of ruminal drinking first showed that D-lactic acidosis existed in neonatal diarrheic calves in the absence of ruminal acidosis. Several studies[25,27,59] have since shown that D-lactic metabolic acidosis is a common occurrence in hospitalized diarrheic calves and that D-lactate concentrations together with occasionally increased L-lactate concentrations largely explain the significantly increased anion gap found in those calves. A study[27] including 300 otherwise unselected calves with neonatal diarrhea admitted to a university hospital found more than half of the calves to have serum D-lactate concentrations higher than 3 mmol/L (**Fig. 3**). In the same study, the subgroup of calves with ruminal acidosis in addition to diarrhea showed significantly higher serum D-lactate concentrations than the calves without ruminal acidosis. However, it was speculated that the ruminal acidosis was not necessarily responsible for the higher D-lactate concentrations. Instead, it was suggested that the ruminal acidosis found in many diarrheic calves was a complication caused by the clinical manifestations of D-lactic acidosis, insofar as the weakness and incoordination caused by increased blood concentrations of

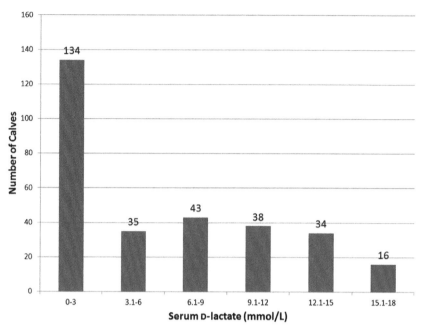

Fig. 3. Serum D-lactate concentrations of 300 calves with neonatal diarrhea. (*From* Lorenz I. Influence of D-lactate on metabolic acidosis and on prognosis in neonatal calves with diarrhoea. J Vet Med A Physiol Pathol Clin Med 2004;51:426; with permission.)

D-lactic acid could interfere with the esophageal groove reflex and thus lead to ruminal drinking.

D-Lactic Metabolic Acidosis in Neonatal Small Ruminants

A syndrome similar to the acidosis without dehydration syndrome in suckler calves was first described in 7 goat kids in 1991.[60] As in calves, this syndrome, now usually referred to as FKD, is characterized by depression and weakness, high anion gap metabolic acidosis, and can be successfully treated with oral or IV therapy with sodium bicarbonate.[60,61] Bleul and colleagues[70] confirmed in 2006 that this syndrome is caused by D-lactic metabolic acidosis. Affected kids do usually not show diarrhea, and the cause of the accumulation of D-lactate remains unclear. Recent reports suggest that the disease can be avoided by hand-rearing kids on cow's milk, milk replacer, or heat-treated milk.[62,63] However, because both studies included only 1 farm each, it is questionable if the results can be generalized.

D-Lactic metabolic acidosis in lambs causing a clinical picture comparable with FKD was first described in 2009.[64] Two neonatal lambs representing a flock problem characterized by somnolence, ataxia or recumbency, and anorexia showed high anion gap acidosis, with base deficit and D-lactate values of 31.9/18.5 mmol/L and 20.1/10.8 mmol/L, respectively. One lamb was in a comatose state at time of admission and was euthanized. The postmortem examination, which included histopathologic examination of the liver, kidneys, spleen, heart, and brain, as well as bacteriologic and parasitologic examinations, showed no abnormalities, with the exception of some oxalate crystals in the renal tubules, which were detected on histopathologic examination. The second lamb recovered after treatment with sodium bicarbonate. Recently, postmortem results of 10 lambs affected by the same syndrome showed different degrees of nephrosis on renal histopathology in all cases.[65] Nephrosis has not been found in any cases of FKD or acidosis without dehydration syndrome. However, not many postmortem results are described in the literature in kids or calves with these disorders, because in all studies, treatment was performed, and in most cases, it was successful. It has also been confirmed in more cases that D-lactic metabolic acidosis in lambs can be treated successfully by application of sodium bicarbonate.[66]

In lambs with mild to moderate diarrhea, serum D-lactate concentrations were increased, but stayed lower than clinically significant concentrations.[67]

TREATMENT OF D-LACTIC METABOLIC ACIDOSIS

Wherever the site of D-lactate production is throughout the gastrointestinal tract, it is obvious that production and absorption of D-lactate can overcome the capacity of metabolism and excretion in calves, goat kids, and lambs to cause these clinical syndromes. This observation implies that successful treatment can either target decrease of D-lactate production and absorption or increase in metabolism and excretion. D-Lactate concentrations decrease regularly within 24 to 48 hours of initiation of therapy that includes correction of acidosis as 1 component.[66,68–70]

Ewaschuk and colleagues[24] considered low kidney perfusion and increased tubular reabsorption of D-lactate in dehydrated calves as the cause of accumulation. Accordingly, enhancement of renal perfusion by rehydration would trigger D-lactate excretion. On first sight, this argument seems to be valid only for diarrheic calves and not the syndromes described that are not accompanied by diarrhea or clinical signs of dehydration. However, because clinical signs of dehydration lag behind the fluid loss, renal perfusion can be impaired in animals without clinically detectable dehydration. Most studies in which urea and creatinine values were reported showed increased urea concentrations in the absence of clinical dehydration either as a mean within the affected group[35,58,70] or individually in most affected animals.[64,65] In 10 calves with diarrhea and dehydration, urine volume and D-lactate clearance increased significantly within the first 6 hours after initiation of IV fluid therapy,[71] which indicates renal excretion as an important factor in the decline of D-lactate concentrations in dehydrated animals.

In addition to rehydration, correction of metabolic acidosis is the other obvious change that may initiate the decline of D-lactate concentration in acidotic diarrheic calves. It can be speculated that production of D-lactate can be influenced by the correction of metabolic acidosis. It seems possible that a vicious cycle with the following elements may develop: lactic acid is formed in the intestine in higher than normal rates, most probably because of malabsorption of carbohydrates in diarrheic calves or dysbacteria of unknown reason, creating an acidic environment in the intestines (intestinal acidosis with a pathogenesis similar to ruminal acidosis). After absorption of lactic acid, the bicarbonate pool is depleted by buffering, and therefore, less bicarbonate is secreted into the intestines; the intestinal environment remains acidic, and lactic acid–forming bacteria are further favored in their multiplication and activity. The cycle could be broken by therapeutic infusion of bicarbonate, and thus, enhancement of bicarbonate secretion into the gut. This theory is supported in a study[71] involving 10 neonatal calves with diarrhea and D-lactic metabolic acidosis in which fecal D-lactate concentrations and fecal pH were measured in quantitatively collected fecal samples in 3-hourly intervals. After correction of the metabolic acidosis within the first 3 hours of the study period, the median of the fecal pH increased from 6.3 to 6.9 in the feces collected over the next 3-hour period. At the same time, the D-lactate concentration and the total mass of excreted D-lactate remained unchanged, but decreased considerable in all samples thereafter.

In humans suffering from short bowel syndrome, different treatment strategies have been tried, but nonspecific therapy for metabolic acidosis with bicarbonate has only seldom been reported in this context. Instead, modification of the abnormal intestinal flora by oral application of antibiotics is the most commonly used therapy.[32] Ewaschuk and colleagues[69] discussed the routine use of antibiotics as 1 possible reason for the decline not only in serum D-lactate but also in fecal D-lactate concentration in diarrheic calves observed after therapy was started. However, the same decline in serum and fecal D-lactate concentration was found in 10 calves after IV fluid therapy and correction of acidosis, whereby only 1 of these calves received antibiotic treatment.[71] A recent study,[72] in which only about half of the involved calves with diarrhea were treated with antibiotics, implied that the complete correction of metabolic acidosis and dehydration are likely to be more important for the treatment success than antibiotic therapy. Because rehydration and correction of acidosis are obviously sufficient for successful treatment of D-lactic metabolic acidosis, and use of antibiotics promotes the selection, and subsequent proliferation, of antibiotic-resistant strains of bacteria, the attempt to reduce D-lactate production by oral antibiotic treatment cannot be recommended for this purpose in neonatal ruminants.

Another common therapeutic strategy in the short bowel syndrome aims at reduction of the quantity of substrate for intestinal fermentation by oral fasting with IV alimentation or change of diet.[32] In newer studies[68,71,72] investigating treatment options for diarrheic calves, milk is usually offered throughout the course of treatment, concurrent with best available scientific evidence, which has shown that withholding milk in calf diarrhea can rapidly lead to malnutrition and emaciation.[73,74] However, because calves are generally severely ill when admitted to university hospitals, most probably, most of the animals involved in these studies experience or will have experienced a period of decreased milk intake when therapy is started, which could also contribute to the declining serum and fecal D-lactate concentrations.

SUPPLEMENTARY DATA

Supplementary data related to this article can be found online at http://dx.doi.org/10.1016/j.cvfa.2014.03.004.

REFERENCES

1. Dunlop RH, Hammond PB. D-lactic acidosis of ruminants. Ann N Y Acad Sci 1965;119(3):1109–32.
2. Omole OO, Brocks DR, Nappert G, et al. High-performance liquid chromatographic assay of (±)-lactic acid and its enantiomers in calf serum. J Chromatogr B Biomed Sci Appl 1999;727(1-2):23–9.
3. Lorenz I, Hartmann I, Gentile A. Determination of D-lactate in calf serum samples–an automated enzymatic assay. Comp Clin Pathol 2003;12(3):169–71.
4. Sousa Silva M, Gomes RA, Ferreira AE, et al. The glyoxalase pathway: the first hundred years... and beyond. Biochem J 2013;453:1–15.
5. Oh MS, Phelps KR, Traube M, et al. D-Lactic acidosis in a man with the short-bowel syndrome. N Engl J Med 1979;301(5):249–52.
6. Tubbs PK. The metabolism of d-alpha hydroxy acids in animal tissues. Ann N Y Acad Sci 1965;119:920–6.
7. Cammack R. Assay, purification and properties of mammalian D-2-hydroxy acid dehydrogenase. Biochem J 1969;115:55–64.

8. Oh MS, Uribarri J, Alveranga D, et al. Metabolic utilization and renal handling of d-lactate in men. Metabolism 1985;34(7):621–5.
9. Giesecke D, Stangassinger M, Henle K. D(-)Milchsäure - ein Stoffwechselproblem. Z Ernahrungswiss 1985;24:172–86 [in German].
10. de Vrese M, Koppenhoefer B, Barth CA. D-lactic acid metabolism after an oral load of dl-lactate. Clin Nutr 1990;9(1):23–8.
11. Flick MJ, Konieczny SF. Identification of putative mammalian d-lactate dehydrogenase enzymes. Biochem Biophys Res Commun 2002;295(4):910–6.
12. Ling B, Peng F, Alcorn J, et al. D-Lactate altered mitochondrial energy production in rat brain and heart but not liver. Nutr Metab 2012;9(1):6.
13. Stangassinger M, Giesecke D. Untersuchungen zur Genese und Biochemie der Pansenacidose. 4. Verteilung von D(-) Milchsäure nach Infusion bei Ziege, Schaf und Rind. Zentralbl Veterinarmed A 1977;24:789–98 [in German].
14. Giesecke D, Stangassinger M. Untersuchungen zur Genese und Biochemie der Pansenacidose. 5. Kinetik der Elimination von D(-)Milchsaure aus dem Blut. Zentralbl Veterinarmed A 1978;25:327–37 [in German].
15. Stangassinger M, Giesecke D. Untersuchungen zur Genese und Biochemie der Pansenacidose. 6. Renale Ausscheidung von Milchsäure-Isomeren. Zentralbl Veterinarmed A 1978;25:597–607 [in German].
16. Klee W. Untersuchungen über die Nierenfunktion bei gesunden und an akutem Durchfall erkrankten Kälbern [Habilitation thesis]. Munich (Germany): University of Munich; 1985 [in German].
17. Lorenz I, Gentile A, Klee W. Investigations of D-lactate metabolism and the clinical signs of D-lactataemia in calves. Vet Rec 2005;156(13):412–5.
18. Dirr L. Untersuchungen über die Dysfunktion des Schlundrinnenreflexes beim jungen Kalb [Doctoral thesis]. Munich (Germany): University of Munich; 1988 [in German].
19. Baur T. Untersuchungen über den Einfluß der intraruminalen Verabreichung von Milch beim jungen Kalb [Doctoral thesis]. Munich (Germany): University of Munich; 1993 [in German].
20. Gentile A. Untersuchungen über die Azidität der Pansenflüssigkeit von Kälbern nach intraruminaler Verabreichung von Rehydratationslösungen. [Acidity of the rumen liquid of calves after intra-ruminal administration of solutions for oral rehydration]. Dtsch Tierarztl Wochenschr 1995;102(6):241–4 [in German].
21. Gentile A, Testoni S, Guglielmini C, et al. Acidosi ruminale cronica nel vitello lattante indotta da somministrazione intraruminale di latte ricostituito. Atti della Società Italiana di Buiatria 1996;28:293–309 [in Italian].
22. Gentile A, Sconza S, Lorenz I, et al. D-Lactic acidosis in calves as a consequence of experimentally induced ruminal acidosis. J Vet Med A Physiol Pathol Clin Med 2004;51(2):64–70.
23. Doll K. Untersuchungen über die Bedeutung unspezifischer Faktoren in der Pathogenese der Diarrhoe beim Kalb [Habilitation thesis]. Munich (Germany): University of Munich; 1992 [in German].
24. Ewaschuk JB, Naylor JM, Palmer R, et al. D-lactate production and excretion in diarrheic calves. J Vet Intern Med 2004;18(5):744–7.
25. Omole OO, Nappert G, Naylor JM, et al. Both L- and D-lactate contribute to metabolic acidosis in diarrheic calves. J Nutr 2001;131(8):2128–31.
26. Grude T. Laktat in Blut, Harn und Pansensaft von Kälbern, insbesondere bei "Pansentrinkern" [Doctoral thesis]. Munich (Germany): University of Munich; 1999 [in German].

27. Lorenz I. Influence of D-lactate on metabolic acidosis and on prognosis in neonatal calves with diarrhoea. J Vet Med A Physiol Pathol Clin Med 2004;51:425–8.
28. Trefz F, Lorch A, Feist M, et al. Metabolic acidosis in neonatal calf diarrhea–clinical findings and theoretical assessment of a simple treatment protocol. J Vet Intern Med 2012;26:162–70.
29. Koch A, Kaske M. Clinical efficacy of intravenous hypertonic saline solution or hypertonic bicarbonate solution in the treatment of inappetent calves with neonatal diarrhea. J Vet Intern Med 2008;22:202–11.
30. König M. Untersuchungen zur Bildung von d-Laktat im Intestinum des Kalbes [Doctoral thesis]. Munich (Germany): University of Munich; 2006 [in German].
31. Bleul U, Fassbind N, Ghielmetti G, et al. Quantitative analysis of fecal flora in goat kids with and without floppy kid syndrome. J Vet Intern Med 2013;27(5): 1283–6.
32. Uribarri J, Oh MS, Carroll HJ. D-lactic acidosis: a review of clinical presentation, biochemical features, and pathophysiologic mechanisms. Medicine (Baltimore) 1998;77(2):73–82.
33. Kasari T, Naylor J. Metabolic acidosis without clinical signs of dehydration in young calves. Can Vet J 1984;25:394–9.
34. Kasari T, Naylor J. Clinical evaluation of sodium bicarbonate, sodium L-lactate and sodium acetate for the treatment of acidosis in diarrheic calves. J Am Vet Med Assoc 1985;187:392–7.
35. Kasari T, Naylor J. Further studies on the clinical features and clinicopathological findings of a syndrome of metabolic acidosis with minimal dehydration in neonatal calves. Can J Vet Res 1986;50:502–8.
36. Naylor J. A retrospective study of the relationship between clinical signs and severity of acidosis in diarrheic calves. Can Vet J 1989;30:577–80.
37. Geishauser T, Thünker B. Metabolische Azidose bei neugeborenen Kälbern mit Durchfall–Abschätzung an Saugreflex oder Stehvermögen. [Metabolic acidosis in diarrheic neonatal calves–estimation using suckling reflex and standing ability]. Prakt Tierarzt 1997;78:600–5 [in German].
38. Wendel H, Sobotka R, Rademacher G. Untersuchungen zur klinischen Abschätzung des Azidosegrades bei Kälbern mit Neugeborenendurchfall. [Study on the correlation between blood acidosis and clinical signs in calves with neonatal diarrhoea]. Tierarztl Umsch 2001;56(7):351–6 [in German].
39. Naylor JM. Severity and nature of acidosis in diarrheic calves over and under one week of age. Can Vet J 1987;28(4):168–73.
40. Lorenz I. Investigations on the influence of serum D-lactate levels on clinical signs in calves with metabolic acidosis. Vet J 2004;168:323–7.
41. Gentile A, Lorenz I, Sconza S, et al. Experimentally induced systemic hyperchloremic acidosis in calves. J Vet Intern Med 2008;22:190–5.
42. Abeysekara S, Naylor JM, Wassef AW, et al. d-Lactic acid-induced neurotoxicity in a calf model. Am J Physiol Endocrinol Metab 2007;293(2):E558–65.
43. Trefz FM, Lorch A, Feist M, et al. The prevalence and clinical relevance of hyperkalaemia in calves with neonatal diarrhoea. Vet J 2013;195(3):350–6.
44. Trefz FM, Constable PD, Sauter-Louis C, et al. Hyperkalemia in neonatal diarrheic calves depends on the degree of dehydration and the cause of the metabolic acidosis but does not require the presence of acidemia. J Dairy Sci 2013; 96(11):7234–44. http://dx.doi.org/10.3168/jds.2013-6945.
45. Cross SA, Callaway CW. D-Lactic acidosis and selected cerebellar ataxias. Mayo Clin Proc 1984;59(3):202–5.

46. Wyss MT, Jolivet R, Buck A, et al. In vivo evidence for lactate as a neuronal energy source. J Neurosci 2011;31(20):7477–85.
47. Gladden LB. Lactate metabolism: a new paradigm for the third millennium. J Physiol 2004;558(1):5–30.
48. Gentile A, Rademacher G, Seemann G, et al. Systemische Auswirkungen der Pansenazidose im Gefolge von Pansentrinken beim Milchkalb: Retrospektive Analyse von 293 Fällen. [Systemic effects of ruminal acidosis following ruminal drinking in young calves: a retrospective analysis of 293 cases]. Tierarztl Prax Ausg G Grosstiere Nutztiere 1998;26G(4):205–9 [in German].
49. Van Bruinessen-Kapsenberg EG, Wensing T, Breukink HJ. Indigestionen der Mastkälber infolge fehlenden Schlundrinnenreflexes. Tierarztl Umsch 1982;37: 515–7.
50. Gentile A, Rademacher G, Klee W. Acidosi ruminale fermentativa nel vitello lattante. Obiettivi e Documenti Veterinari 1997;18(12):63–75 [in Italian].
51. Dirksen G, Dirr L. Oesophageal groove dysfunction as a complication of neonatal diarrhea in the calf. Bov Pract 1989;24:53–60.
52. Rademacher G, Korn N, Friedrich A. Der Pansentrinker als Patient in der Praxis. Tierarztl Umsch 2003;58:115–25 [in German].
53. Doll K. "Trinkschwäche"/Anorexie beim neugeborenen Kalb: Ursachen, Folgen und Behandlung. Prakt Tierarzt 1990;72(Collegium Vet. XXI):16–8 [in German].
54. van Weeren-Keverling Buisman A. Ruminal drinking in veal calves. Utrecht (The Netherlands): Proefschrift; 1989.
55. Dirksen G, Baur T. Force-feeding and rumen acidosis in young calves. Bov Pract 1990;25:29–33.
56. Rademacher G, Friedrich A. Untersuchungen zur Prognose von Kälbern mit Pansenazidose infolge Pansentrinkens. Tierarztl Umsch 2003;58:63–70 [in German].
57. Stocker H, Lutz H, Kaufmann C, et al. Acid-base disorders in milk fed calves with chronic indigestion. Vet Rec 1999;145:340–6.
58. Schelcher F, Marcillaud S, Braun J, et al. Metabolic acidosis without dehydration and no or minimal diarrhoea in suckler calves is caused by hyper-D-lactatemia. Proceedings of the XX. World Buiatrics Congress. Sydney, July 6–10, 1998. p. 371–4.
59. Ewaschuk J, Naylor J, Zello G. Anion gap correlates with serum D- and DL-lactate concentration in diarrheic neonatal calves. J Vet Intern Med 2003;17:940–2.
60. Tremblay RR, Butler DG, Allen JW, et al. Metabolic acidosis without dehydration in seven goat kids. Can Vet J 1991;32(5):308.
61. Gufler H, Pernthaner A. "Neonatales Lähmungssyndrom" bei Ziegenkitzen: Folge einer metabolischen Azidose. ["Neonatal paretic syndrome" in goat kids: a result of metabolic acidosis]. Wien Tierarztl Monatsschr 1999;86(11): 382–9 [in German].
62. Gufler H. Prevention of floppy kid syndrome: a long-term clinical field study conducted on a goat farm in South Tyrol/Italy. Small Rumin Res 2012;108(1–3): 113–9.
63. Klein C, Bostedt H, Wehrend A. D-lactate elevation as a cause of metabolic acidosis in newborn goat kids–the potential role of milk ingestion as etiopathogenetic factor. Tierarztl Prax 2010;38:371–6.
64. Lorenz I, Lorch A. D-lactic acidosis in lambs. Vet Rec 2009;164:174–5.
65. Angell JW, Jones G, Grove-White DH, et al. A prospective on farm cohort study investigating the epidemiology and pathophysiology of drunken lamb syndrome. Vet Rec 2013;172(6):154.

66. Angell JW, Jones GL, Voigt K, et al. Successful correction of D-lactic acid neurotoxicity (drunken lamb syndrome) by bolus administration of oral sodium bicarbonate. Vet Rec 2013;173(8):193.

67. Saman Abeysekara AW. D-lactic acid metabolism and control of acidosis [thesis]. Saskatoon (Canada): University of Saskatchewan; 2009.

68. Lorenz I, Vogt S. Investigations on the association of D-lactate blood concentrations with the outcome of therapy of acidosis, and with posture and demeanour in young calves with diarrhoea. J Vet Med A Physiol Pathol Clin Med 2006;53: 490–4.

69. Ewaschuk JB, Zello GA, Naylor JM. *Lactobacillus* GG does not affect D-lactic acidosis in diarrheic calves, in a clinical setting. J Vet Intern Med 2006;20(3): 614–9.

70. Bleul U, Schwantag S, Stocker H, et al. Floppy kid syndrome caused by D-lactic acidosis in goat kids. J Vet Intern Med 2006;20(4):1003–8.

71. Reischer N. Dynamik der Serumkonzentration und Ausscheidung von D-Laktat bei jungen Kälbern mit Durchfall [Doctoral thesis]. Munich (Germany): University of Munich; 2012 [in German].

72. Trefz F, Lorch A, Feist M, et al. Construction and validation of a decision tree for treating metabolic acidosis in calves with neonatal diarrhea. BMC Vet Res 2012; 8(1):238.

73. Heath SE, Naylor JM, Guedo BL, et al. The effects of feeding milk to diarrheic calves supplemented with oral electrolytes. Can J Vet Res 1989;53:477–85.

74. Garthwaite BD, Drackley JK, McCoy GC, et al. Whole milk and oral rehydration solution for calves with diarrhea of spontaneous origin. J Dairy Sci 1994;77: 835–43.

Sodium Balance and the Dysnatremias

Stacey R. Byers, DVM, MS*, Andrea S. Lear, DVM, David C. Van Metre, DVM

KEYWORDS

- Sodium balance • Dysnatremias • Hypernatremia • Hyponatremia

KEY POINTS

- The serum sodium concentration is expressed as the quantity of sodium divided by the volume of water in the serum.
- Disorders of sodium concentration often reflect disorders in water homeostasis.
- Hypernatremia most commonly occurs when there is a sustained loss of water from the body, or when an animal ingests or is force-fed a sodium-rich fluid without adequate amounts of free (pure) water.
- Hyponatremia most commonly occurs when an animal loses sodium and water in diarrhea or in urine with ingestion or retention of only water, resulting in dilution of the extracellular fluid sodium concentration.
- When treating severe hypernatremia or hyponatremia, it is most prudent for the veterinarian to correct these disorders slowly to avoid potentially serious neurologic complications.

INTRODUCTION

The dysnatremias are defined as abnormalities in serum sodium concentration.[1] Depending on the magnitude and duration of the sodium abnormality and the nature of any concurrent or primary disease, hypernatremia and hyponatremia may result in no consequences, subclinical impairment of health and productivity, or severe clinical disease. Dysnatremias can be the sequelae to diseases or environmental conditions that promote fluid gain or loss from the body, as well as medical interventions that add excessive amounts of sodium or water to the extracellular fluid (ECF). Extreme, sustained dysnatremia may result in central nervous system (CNS) dysfunction and death.

The authors have nothing to disclose.
Department of Clinical Sciences, College of Veterinary Medicine and Biomedical Sciences, Colorado State University, Fort Collins, CO 80523-1620, USA
* Corresponding author.
E-mail address: stacey.byers@colostate.edu

Vet Clin Food Anim 30 (2014) 333–350
http://dx.doi.org/10.1016/j.cvfa.2014.03.003

SERUM SODIUM CONCENTRATION AND OSMOLARITY

The sodium concentration of the ECF is accurately represented by the serum sodium concentration. This concentration can be viewed in the same light as a fraction is viewed in mathematics, with the numerator the sodium concentration and the denominator the volume of serum water. In most ruminant species, the normal range of serum sodium concentration is approximately 135 to 155 mEq/L.[2] In New World camelids (NWCs), the normal range of serum sodium concentration is slightly higher, at 147 to 158 mEq/L.[3]

When the ECF sodium concentration is abnormal, the normal animal restores normal serum sodium concentration (eunatremia) by increasing or decreasing the amount of the water in the body. Because regulation of sodium concentration is based on the body's management of water, dysnatremias can be thought of as disorders of water balance.[4,5] It is vital that the clinician thinks of sodium concentration not as an indicator of the amount of sodium in the ECF, but rather as the relative ratio of sodium to water.

Sodium is the predominant cation in the ECF. Sodium and its accompanying anions are the solutes that exert the greatest influence on osmolarity of the ECF.[6] Osmolarity is the concentration of particles per liter of water. Almost all cellular membranes are highly permeable to water, so a disparity of osmolarity between the intracellular fluid (ICF) and ECF results in rapid movement of water from the fluid compartment with low osmolarity to that of higher osmolarity. When an osmotic gradient exists between the ECF and ICF, the ensuing movement of water results in cellular shrinkage or swelling. Therefore, osmolarity is tightly controlled to prevent potentially detrimental changes in cellular volume.[7,8]

The osmolarity of the ECF is accurately represented by a serum sample and can be measured in the laboratory with an osmometer. In most animals, normal serum osmolality (for dilute fluids such as the ECF, osmolarity [expressed as mOsm/L] and osmolality [expressed as mOsm/kg] are approximately equal and are essentially synonymous[6]) ranges from approximately 270 to 310 mOsm/kg.[9] This result is commonly referred to as the measured osmolarity. Osmometers require frequent calibration and intensive maintenance and are not commonly available in private practices, so the calculated serum osmolarity is more commonly used. Serum osmolarity is estimated using the following equation[10]:

$$\text{Serum osmolarity} = (2 \times [\text{Na}^+]) + \frac{[\text{glucose}]}{18} + \frac{\text{BUN}}{2.8}$$

where serum [Na$^+$] is expressed in mEq/L and serum [glucose] and blood urea nitrogen [BUN] are expressed in mg/dL and the result is referred to as the calculated osmolarity.

The difference between the measured and calculated osmolarity is termed the osmolar gap. In most healthy animals, the osmolar gap is less than 10 mOsm/L. An osmolar gap greater than this value may indicate 1 or more of the following[10]:

1. Laboratory error in osmometry or serum biochemistry
2. True states of decreased ECF water content caused by severe hyperlipemia or hyperproteinemia or
3. The presence of unmeasured, low-molecular-weight solutes in the serum, such as ethylene glycol or ethanol

Ethylene glycol intoxication has been reported in livestock.[11,12] It is characterized by hyperosmolarity, an increased osmolar gap, metabolic acidosis, azotemia, hypocalcemia, and a high case fatality rate.

PHYSIOLOGIC REGULATION OF ECF OSMOLARITY AND VOLUME

Osmolarity is controlled primarily through mechanisms that adjust the amount of water in which solutes such as sodium are suspended. Homeostasis of osmolarity is simplistically viewed as water driven. Thirst (water ingestion) and water retention by the kidney are mechanisms by which water can be retained in the body. Alternatively, a lack of thirst and elimination of water by the kidney allow water to be lost from the body.

Variations in ECF osmolarity trigger different effector responses. Increased osmolarity initiates the sensation of thirst, the release of antidiuretic hormone (ADH), which limits water losses in urine.[13] Decreased ECF osmolarity occurs when water enters the ECF without a proportionate entry of sodium, for example, with excessive water ingestion. In the normal animal, reduction of ECF osmolarity causes inhibition of the thirst response and inhibition of ADH release, thus producing dilute, water-rich urine.[13]

The ECF volume is regulated by physiologic mechanisms that control retention and excretion of sodium; therefore, volume homeostasis can be simplistically viewed as sodium driven. These mechanisms include the autonomic nervous system, the renin-angiotensin-aldosterone system (RAAS), and atrial natriuretic peptide (ANP). These volume-regulating responses do not generate significant changes in the sodium concentration of the ECF, because as sodium is moved into or out of the ECF, there is a concurrent, parallel, and proportionate movement of water.[14] Hypovolemia triggers circulatory mechanoreceptors, resulting in rapid activation of the sympathetic nervous system, which increases reabsorption of sodium and chloride ions in the kidneys.[15] Reduced distension pressure in the nephron initiates RAAS through renin release from the cells of the juxtaglomerular apparatus. The RAAS cascade results in the production of angiotensin II, which increases the efficiency of sodium and water retention by the nephron and activates aldosterone release from the adrenal glands.[15] Aldosterone enhances sodium reclamation from the nephrons, gastrointestinal (GI) tract, and salivary gland, resulting in water following sodium into the ECF.[16] Salt hunger and thirst are stimulated by hypovolemia, and these responses aid by prompting addition of sodium and water to the body.

Hypervolemia activates similar but opposing pathways. A reduction in sympathetic tone to the kidney results in diminished sodium, chloride, and water reclamation. The RAAS is not activated. Hypervolemia induces increased perfusion pressure to the kidney and an increase in the glomerular filtration rate (GFR), which drives tubular fluid through the nephron and results in increased elimination in the urine, a phenomenon termed pressure diuresis.[15] Hypervolemia also causes stretching of the cardiac atria, triggering release of ANP, which also increases GFR and inhibits sodium reabsorption. Natriuresis and diuresis follow.[17] In the CNS, ANP seems to directly inhibit salt hunger and thirst. These responses collectively serve to reduce increased ECF volume and restore euvolemia.

WATER REQUIREMENTS

Daily water requirements for small ruminants and cattle have been published.[18–20] Milk and milk replacers provide water and variable amounts of sodium for the neonate. Whole milk typically has less than 17 mEq/L of sodium, whereas milk replacers have 60 to 80 mEq/L.[21,22]

CLASSIFICATION OF THE DYSNATREMIAS

In the medical literature, hypernatremia and hyponatremia are commonly described as either acute or chronic; however, it is often difficult to accurately determine the duration of dysnatremia.[21,23] Livestock owners may be unable to discern the onset of disease with sufficient accuracy to enable the veterinarian to classify the disorder by its duration. In addition, the onset of the dysnatremia may not necessarily coincide with the onset of the primary medical problem. These problems limit the relevance of classifying the dysnatremias by their duration. However, the duration and severity of the dysnatremia can profoundly affect osmotic homeostasis within brain cells, with potentially critical clinical implications.[24] Because of the pathophysiologic relevance of the duration of dysnatremia and the commonality of this classification scheme in the literature, it is discussed in this review.

HYPERNATREMIA

In livestock and NWCs, the risk for hypernatremia is highest in the following situations:

1. Sustained water loss occurs as a result of panting, water deprivation, evaporative losses from burns, or diuresis induced by persistent hyperglycemia.
2. Oral or parenteral, sodium-containing crystalloid solutions are administered to an animal without access to free water, or that is unable to ingest free water.
3. An animal ingests a sodium-containing salt without ingesting an adequate volume of water to balance the sodium load.

Livestock can tolerate ingestion of large quantities of sodium (≤13% of dry matter intake) provided that ad libitum access to palatable and pure (relatively sodium-free) water is allowed.[25] High-sodium feedstuffs include whey, bakery waste, salted fish products, and certain by-products of the restaurant industry. Improperly formulated electrolyte replacement solutions, liquid mineral supplements, and milk replacers are a common source of excess sodium for confined livestock. Environmental sources of sodium for pastured livestock include effluent from petroleum drills, well water from basins with high soil sodium content, and seawater in tidal marshes. In the absence of a source of pure water, ingestion of water containing a sodium chloride concentration of approximately 1% or higher consistently results in sodium intoxication (salt poisoning).[25]

Based on a few published reports,[25] subclinical salt intoxication is manifested as reduced productivity and impaired fertility. Presumably, clinical signs of sodium intoxication are avoided in these animals because they subsequently acquire access to pure water.

Acute Hypernatremia

Although there is no clear consensus in the literature as to what time frame defines acute intoxication, hypernatremia that develops within 48 hours has been proposed.[24,26]

When large quantities of sodium are ingested without adequate water, diarrhea develops within hours as a result of the high osmotic load in the GI tract as well as direct chemical irritation of the mucosa. Mucus and blood may be evident in the feces. CNS dysfunction has been attributed to the resultant rapid dehydration and shrinkage of brain cells. High intracellular sodium content disrupts neuronal energy metabolism and normal intracellular ionic gradients.[25–27] Nervous signs are variable and include aimless wandering, head pressing, obtundation, blindness, tetraparesis, tremors, ataxia, recumbency, opisthotonus, and seizures (**Fig. 1**). Fasciculation of the facial muscles has been noticed in some cases.[26] Death occurs as a result of centrally mediated respiratory failure.

Differential diagnoses for acute sodium intoxication include polioencephalomalacia, lead intoxication, head trauma, meningitis (including rabies), nervous ketosis,

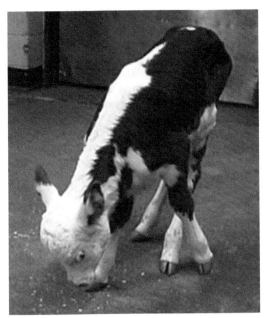

Fig. 1. Calf with neurologic signs of hypernatremia, including head pressing, tremors, and fasciculation of the facial muscles. (*Courtesy of* Dr Geof Smith, North Carolina State University, Raleigh, NC.)

nervous coccidiosis, hypomagnesemia, hypocalcemia, grass staggers syndromes (eg, ryegrass), pregnancy toxemia, and in small ruminants, focal symmetric encephalomalacia caused by *Clostridium perfringens* type D. In neonates, hypernatremia may accompany a multitude of primary disorders, because impairment of water or milk ingestion can limit the animal's ability to compensate for both insensible water losses.

The severity of the accompanying hypernatremia is dependent on the timing of sampling relative to ingestion, the quantity of sodium ingested, and the volume, if any, of water ingested by the animal. Typically, the cerebrospinal fluid (CSF) sodium concentration increases to greater than 160 mEq/L.[25] The ratio of CSF sodium to serum sodium may be greater than 1.[25]

Case example
On a 4500-head commercial sheep ranch in southeastern Wyoming, a 4-year-old, lactating female crossbreed sheep was examined for evaluation of recumbency and obtunded mentation of 8 hours duration. A second ewe had shown similar signs earlier that day and had died without treatment; the carcass was not available for examination. The ewe had given birth to 2 healthy lambs 17 days before the onset of illness. The ewe was one of 30 ewes and 54 lambs that had been moved into a 10-acre, fenced-in grass pasture on the previous evening. The ewes were immunized annually for tetanus and *C perfringens* types C and D, with the most recent booster immunization having been administered 2 months previously.

Before being moved onto pasture, the ewes and lambs had been kept in a lambing corral for approximately 14 days. While in the lambing corral, the ewes and lambs were provided ad libitum grass hay and water, which was pumped into troughs from a nearby stream. The pasture onto which the sheep had been moved contained a mixture of native grasses and shrubs; access to the same stream was provided at a corner of the pasture. A feeder containing a sodium chloride block was present in the center of the pasture. The sodium chloride block was not supplemented with trace minerals or medications. A fenced-in enclosure with a shed was present in the center of the pasture, and the ewes and lambs had been moved into the enclosure on the previous evening and confined there overnight for approximately 12 hours. Both affected ewes had been found recumbent within this enclosure. The enclosure included straw bedding but had no water or salt within it.

Inspection of the pasture showed no toxic plants or materials. Physical examination of the affected ewe showed recumbency, flaccid tetraparesis, and a severely obtunded demeanor (**Fig. 2**). Heart rate, respiratory rate, and rectal temperature were normal, as were hydration status, mucous membrane color, and capillary refill time. Neurologic examination showed fasciculations of the facial muscles and variable, intermittent, bilateral nystagmus. Vision, pupillary light responses, muscle tone, and spinal reflexes were normal. The ewe's blood glucose concentration, as determined by a portable glucometer, was 404 mg/dL (normal, 70–100). Differential diagnoses were listeriosis, bacterial meningitis, rabies, salt intoxication/water deprivation, *C perfringens* type D enterotoxemia, and head trauma. The producer was informed of the differential diagnoses and case management options and chose diagnostic testing to determine the cause of the problem as well as treatment of the ewe. Venous blood samples were obtained for hematologic and biochemical analysis. A sample of CSF was obtained by lumbosacral puncture. Dexamethasone (0.5 mg/kg intravenously [IV]), oxytetracycline (11 mg/kg IV), and *C perfringens* types C and D antitoxin (20 mL subcutaneously [SC]) were administered. The ewe died approximately 30 minutes after treatment was initiated.

The ewe was submitted for necropsy. Fluorescent antibody testing of brain tissue for rabies virus was negative. Gross necropsy showed multiple mediastinal abscesses suggestive of caseous lymphadenitis. Serum biochemical analysis showed hypernatremia (195 mEq/L; normal, 142–152), hyperchloremia (152 mEq/L; normal, 103–113), and hyperglycemia (419 mg/dL). All other biochemical and hematologic parameters were within normal limits. Analysis of CSF showed no cytologic abnormalities.

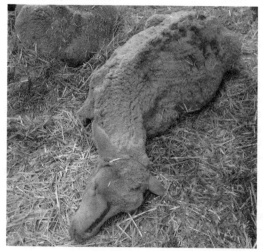

Fig. 2. Recumbent ewe with neurologic signs resulting from hypernatremia.

However, the sodium concentration of the CSF was 196 mEq/L (normal, <160), and the CSF/serum sodium ratio was greater than 1, suggestive of salt intoxication. Histologic examination of cerebrum, cerebellum, and brainstem showed perivascular edema and occasional perivascular hemorrhage. The sodium concentration of brain tissue was 10,500 ppm (normal, 5500–5700 ppm). A diagnosis of acute sodium intoxication was made, with the internal form of caseous lymphadenitis considered a coincidental finding.

The shepherd responsible for the affected group of ewes was interviewed. On the evening before the onset of signs in the 2 ewes, the shepherd had moved the group from the lambing corral into the grass pasture. The shepherd observed several ewes vigorously ingesting the block of salt; however, he had subsequently moved the ewes into the overnight enclosure without allowing the animals to have access to water. Apparently, the affected ewe had voluntarily ingested sufficient amounts of salt to induce acute sodium intoxication. Loss of free water from the ewe's ECF space likely occurred through insensible losses and lactation. The hyperglycemia detected was considered to indicate a stress response.

Given that the ewes had been allowed access to ad libitum hay and water only while being held in a corral for 2 weeks, it is likely that significant salt hunger had developed. To correct this problem, salt supplementation of the flock was initiated in all corrals and pastures, and salt sources were relocated near water supplies in all pastures. No additional cases occurred.

Iatrogenic acute hypernatremia

Multiple cases of iatrogenic salt intoxication have been reported secondary to feeding improperly formulated oral electrolyte solutions to diarrheic neonates.[21,28,29] Addition of excessive quantities of electrolyte powder to an inadequate volume of water is the typical error, followed by force-feeding of the solution via orogastric tube to the ill neonate. Homemade electrolyte replacement formulas may also contain excessive amounts of sodium.[26] Affected neonates may not compensate for the sodium load by drinking milk or water, either because of unavailability or the primary illness limited the neonate's capacity to drink or suckle.

Ollivet and McGuirk[22] reported salt intoxication in a herd of dairy calves that was caused by multiple factors: (1) the use of high salinity well water to prepare milk replacer; (2) addition of additional milk replacer powder to the prescribed volume of water on the milk replacer label, presumably to add additional nutrients during cold weather; (3) mixing of oral electrolytes directly into milk replacer; and (4) a lack availability of pure water for the calves.

Iatrogenic, acute hypernatremia also occurs as a result of resuscitation therapy with hypertonic (7.2%) saline solution.[30] The resuscitative effect of hypertonic fluid therapy is caused by an acute shift of water from the intracellular space to the ECF and bloodstream, thereby augmenting perfusion to vital organs. The hypernatremia that results from hypertonic sodium-containing resuscitation fluids is rendered transient through provision of free water by drinking or orogastric administration, or by isotonic parenteral fluid therapy.

Spontaneous acute hypernatremia

Spontaneous hypernatremia has been reported in a few diarrheic calves that were not fed oral electrolytes.[29] It was hypothesized that water losses in diarrhea had exceeded fecal sodium losses in these cases, resulting in a relatively greater depletion of ECF water than of sodium (hypotonic fluid loss).[31] Insensible water losses from the respiratory tract could also have contributed to this condition.

Chronic Hypernatremia

Chronic hypernatremia has been defined as hypernatremia that develops gradually over a 4-day to 7-day period.[32,33] The same factors that contribute to acute hypernatremia are at play in chronic hypernatremia (ie, sustained free water losses from the ECF occur, or sodium enters the ECF without proportionate entry of water). The magnitude of hypernatremia can be identical between the acute and chronic forms, and the clinical signs are identical. The 2 conditions are distinguished solely by the rate of increase in serum sodium concentration and the duration that the condition exists.

The primary pathologic distinction between acute and chronic hypernatremia is that in the latter instance, the brain cells undergo biochemical changes to match the osmolarity of brain cytoplasm with that of the high ECF osmolarity. The brain cells increase the intracellular sodium concentration and generate novel intracellular organic solutes, termed idiogenic osmoles, to help retain intracellular water. These organic solutes include myoinositol, betaine, phosphocreatine, glutamine, and glutamate.[33] This adaptation reduces water egress from the cytoplasm of brain cells under sustained hyperosmolar stress, thereby maintaining intracellular hydration and preventing lethal cell shrinkage.

The pathologic consequence of the brain's adjustment to chronic hypernatremia becomes evident if the patient undergoes rapid rehydration, with a lower sodium concentration fluid resulting in a rapid reduction of ECF osmolarity. Movement of water across the osmolar gradient from the ECF into brain cells creates potentially fatal cerebral edema.[33] The veterinary literature refers to this condition as salt poisoning/water intoxication caused by the pathophysiologic role of sudden water entry into the ECF and subsequent movement into the relatively hyperosmolar brain cells.[25]

Hypernatremia Associated with Persistent Hyperglycemia

Hypernatremia associated with persistent hyperglycemia has been described in NWCs.[34,35] Although iatrogenic hyperglycemia has been associated with corticosteroid administration and overzealous IV administration of glucose-containing solutions, most cases of hyperglycemia in NWCs develop secondary to the animal's response to a primary disease process[36] or stressful event.[37] NWCs typically have low circulating insulin concentrations and are relatively insulin resistant.[37] These nuances of energy metabolism become clinically apparent when disorders arise that further antagonize the release or peripheral effects of insulin. Hyperglycemia greater than 400 mg/dL in NWCs occurs, and some affected crias have developed serum glucose concentrations in excess of 1300 mg/dL.[34,35]

Because glucose is an osmotically active solute, hyperglycemia affects the ECF concentration of sodium by influencing the movement of water into and out of the ECF. Initially, hyperglycemia promotes water efflux from the ICF into the ECF, and serum sodium concentration may transiently decline as this water dilutes the sodium. If hyperglycemia is severe enough to exceed the renal threshold in camelids (postulated to be approximately 200 mg/dL),[37] glucose spillover into the urine creates concomitant free water loss in urine, as a result of the electrochemical attraction between glucose and water.[34,35] This loss of water from the ECF depletes the serum sodium concentration of its denominator, resulting in hypernatremia. A serum sodium concentration of greater than 170 mg/dL in hyperglycemic NWCs may indicate risk of subsequent CNS dysfunction.[37] Affected NWCs may develop ataxia, obtundation, head tremors, opisthotonus, and seizures. Polyuria is seen, and glucosuria is evident on urinalysis. The mechanism of CNS dysfunction is unknown, but, as in other species, neuronal dehydration from water efflux or excessive sodium entry into brain cells could be involved. Activation of the RAAS promotes sodium and water retention in the ECF, but the continued loss of water through glucose diuresis worsens the hypernatremic state.[37] In NWCs, this syndrome of variable CNS dysfunction with concurrent hypernatremia, hyperglycemia, and osmotic diuresis from glucosuria has been termed the hyperosmolar syndrome.[34,35]

HYPONATREMIA

Hyponatremia typically results from the addition of water (the denominator) to the ECF without a proportionate addition of sodium (the numerator).[4,5] Hyponatremia, therefore, is a state of relative water excess in the ECF. In livestock and NWCs, the risk of hyponatremia is highest in the following situations:

1. Sodium, other electrolytes, and water are lost from the body in diarrhea and are replaced by ingestion of water.[38–40]
2. Sodium, other electrolytes, and water are lost from the body in renal disease and are replaced by ingestion of water or by retention of water in the ECF along with retained solutes (eg, urea).[41–47]
3. Sodium moves from the ECF into a body cavity or is sequestered in the dysfunctional GI tract (so-called third-space movement of sodium).[23]

Acute Hyponatremia

Acute hyponatremia is defined as hyponatremia that develops within 48 hours.[23] Most commonly, acute hyponatremia results from loss of water and sodium from the body, with subsequent replacement of only water. The resulting dysnatremia has been termed dilutional hyponatremia.[23] Depending on the rate of loss of sodium-rich fluid in diarrhea and the amount of water ingested in compensation, the hyponatremic animal may be euvolemic or hypovolemic.

In 22 cases of acute renal disease in cattle, hyponatremia was present in 14 (63%) and hypochloremia was present in 19 (86%).[48] Solutes that are retained in renal failure, such as urea, may contribute to water retention in the body, contributing to hyponatremia.[23]

Acute hyponatremia can also occur if sodium moves into third-space locations (ie, body cavities or the lumen of the bowel).[23] A common example is urinary tract obstruction that causes secondary bladder rupture and uroperitoneum. The urine liberated into the abdominal cavity contains low concentrations of sodium and chloride relative to the ECF. Therefore, sodium and chloride diffuse from the ECF into the abdominal cavity.[49] Urine contains a variety of solutes excreted as waste products and is hyperosmolar relative to the ECF. During uroperitoneum, those solutes pull ECF water into the abdominal cavity, causing hypovolemia and clinical signs of dehydration.[49]

Uncommon causes of hyponatremia include the following conditions:

- Primary (psychogenic) polydipsia[7,23,26]
- Congestive heart failure[23,26]
- Hemorrhage[23,26]
- The syndrome of inappropriate ADH release (SIADH) (excessive ADH release from neoplastic cells or brain cells) has yet to be reported in livestock and NWCs. In human patients with SIADH, hyponatremia results from excessive water retention by the kidney.[4,7]
- Administration of large volumes of sodium-free or sodium-depleted parenteral fluids, such as 5% dextrose or 0.45% NaCl/2.5% dextrose.

- Sustained exercise in endurance athletes, with losses of water and sodium occurring through profuse sweating; fluid replacement with only water can contribute.[50]
- Nonexertional heat stroke associated with hot weather.[51,52]
- The loss of solutes (including sodium) exceeds the apparent loss of water from the body (in feces, sweat, or urine), termed hypertonic fluid loss.[31]
- Administration of mannitol may dilute serum sodium sufficiently to cause hyponatremia.[7] This process has been termed translocational hyponatremia.[23] Translocational hyponatremia may also result from acute hyperglycemia of iatrogenic, dietary, or pathologic origin.
- Pseudohyponatremia is a laboratory artifact that can occur if severe hyperproteinemia or hyperlipidemia is present and if flame photometry is used to measure serum sodium concentration.[4,7]

Clinical signs of acute hyponatremia

Specific clinical signs of acute hyponatremia have not been well defined in livestock and camelids.[26,30,38] In diarrheic neonates, hypoglycemia, metabolic acidosis, and hyperkalemia may also exist concurrently.[39,40,53,54] The weakness, ataxia, and obtundation that these metabolic derangements produce can overlap with any clinical signs that might be caused by hyponatremia.

In humans, clinical signs of moderate, acute hyponatremia (serum Na^+ level = 125–129 mEq/L) are nonspecific and include nausea, vomiting, confusion, disorientation, and headache.[7] In humans, severe, acute hyponatremia (serum Na^+ level <125 mEq/L) may result in more serious neurologic signs,[23] particularly if hyponatremia develops rapidly (a reduction in serum Na^+ level >0.5 mEq/L/h).[55] Cerebral edema occurs and may result in seizures, coma, respiratory arrest, and death. This condition is rare in humans and usually results from self-intoxication with water in individuals with psychological disorders or as a rare, idiopathic complication of surgery.[23] Wong and colleagues[56] reported a case of severe hyponatremia (105 mEq/L) with neurologic signs in a foal with a 24-hour history of acute diarrhea.

Chronic Hyponatremia

Hyponatremia that develops over a period of 48 hours or more has been designated as chronic hyponatremia.[7] In response to sustained hypo-osmolarity in the ECF, brain cells adapt by losing electrolytes and organic solutes from their intracellular space. In so doing, the brain cells are able to limit changes in cell volume.

Potentially serious sequelae occur if the patient ingests large quantities of salt or is administered sodium-rich fluids orally or parenterally. Rapid sodium entry into the ECF creates an osmotic gradient favoring rapid water egress from the neurons. In humans and laboratory animals, this pathologic process is manifested by bilaterally symmetric demyelination of neurons in the pons, thalamus, and other sites in the brain, a process termed central pontine neurolysis or osmotic demyelination syndrome (ODS).[7,23,57] Typically, in affected humans, initial signs of encephalopathy abate with correction of hyponatremia; however, 2 to 5 days after treatment, progressive ataxia, dysphagia, myoclonus, spastic tetraparesis, and death may ensue.[23,57] Although reports of severe neurologic disease after correction of chronic hyponatremia have been reported in horses, lesions of ODS were not found.[56,58] Lesions compatible with ODS have been described in severely hyponatremic dogs undergoing corrective fluid therapy, with characteristic thalamic lesions detected by magnetic resonance imaging.[59] ODS has not been described in livestock or camelids.

TREATMENT

There is no clear consensus in the medical or veterinary medical literature regarding the optimal treatment of dysnatremias. In our opinion, this lack of consensus may reflect the difficulty in establishing the duration of dysnatremia and disparate definitions of the severity of these disorders. Accurate answers for the following questions would provide the clinician with the clearest path to select the most appropriate treatment of the dysnatremias:

1. Pending measurement of the patient's serum sodium concentration, can the risk of dysnatremia be identified through signalment, history, and physical examination?
2. Can measurement of the serum sodium concentration be obtained promptly?
3. If dysnatremia exists, and is subjectively judged to be mild, moderate, or severe, can the clinician discern the duration that the dysnatremia has existed?
4. Can the clinician discern the rate at which serum sodium concentration has changed over the course of the disease?
5. Is the dysnatremia the primary clinical problem, or is it a sequela of another disease process?

In many scenarios encountered in livestock practice, prompt measurement of serum sodium concentration in the patient is inconsistently available. Nonetheless, pretreatment measurement of sodium and other electrolytes, as well as blood pH and glucose, is ideal.[29] Optimal critical care of the chronically or severely dysnatremic patient requires frequent, serial measurement of serum sodium concentration during fluid therapy, with meticulous adjustment of fluid therapy to ensure gradual restoration of eunatremia.[23,57] This might be an impractical intensive care situation for the busy livestock practitioner in the field or practice setting, and therefore, referral to an intensive care facility may be warranted. For all patients, the environmental effects on salt and water balance should be considered during treatment (eg, shade, fans, and cool sand bedding are helpful in lessening insensible water losses).

For most animals undergoing appropriate IV fluid therapy, if no underlying neurologic disease is present, restoration of euvolemia and perfusion of the kidney is expected to result in some degree of noticeable improvement in the patient's mentation. If the patient's neurologic status deteriorates in the face of fluid therapy, the potential for brain swelling or shrinkage or ODS should be considered.[4,26] Fluid therapy should then be discontinued, and serum and CSF sodium concentrations should be measured. The serum sodium concentration may have been partially or completely corrected by the time these neurologic signs develop. Serum pH, glucose, calcium, potassium, and magnesium concentrations should also be evaluated. Treatment of cerebral edema should be initiated if CSF sodium analysis or ruling out other conditions makes dysnatremia the most likely cause of the animal's neurologic signs.

Table 1 provides information regarding the sodium concentration of several IV fluids used for the treatment of hypernatremia and hyponatremia, as discussed in the following sections.

Fluid Therapy for Acute Hypernatremia (<48 hours)

In acute hypernatremia, the brain cells of the patient have not developed idiogenic osmoles. This situation explains the success that many have reported with the use of either isotonic, sodium-containing or polyionic fluid therapy at a rate that reflects maintenance needs plus any ongoing losses. Fluids used for this purpose include isotonic (0.9%) saline, lactated Ringer solution (LRS), or other products with

Table 1
Sodium concentration of common commercially available IV fluids

Fluid	Na$^+$ Concentration (mEq/L)
0.9% saline	154
Lactated Ringer solution	130
Plasma-Lyte A[a]	140
Normosol-R[b]	140
Isotonic (1.3%) sodium bicarbonate	156
Hypertonic (1.4%) sodium bicarbonate	167
Hypertonic (7.2%) saline	1232

[a] Plasma-Lyte A, Baxter Healthcare, Deerfield, IL.
[b] Normosol-R, Hospira, Lake Forest, IL.

intermediate sodium concentrations (see **Table 1**). Although rapid correction of acute hypernatremia has been accomplished successfully, the consensus across the medical and veterinary medical literature favors a gradual correction plan, with careful monitoring of the patient's neurologic status.[4,7,21,23,26,57]

Bolus fluid therapy may be ideal for animals for which continuous IV fluid therapy is difficult, such as neonates housed with their dams. For NWCs with acute hypernatremia, Cebra[38] recommends an initial IV bolus of 2% of the animal's body weight (BW), or 4% if dehydration is evident. Often, there is concurrent hypoalbuminemia increasing the risk of pulmonary edema in the patient if administered a large bolus of IV fluid. Therefore, when sustained IV fluid therapy is an option for the hypernatremic NWC, 5% of the animal's BW of a polyionic, isotonic, sodium-containing fluid should be administered over a 24-hour period.[38]

The amount of water needed to be administered to the acutely hypernatremic patient can be estimated using the following formula[1]:

$$\text{Liters of water} = 0.6 \times (\text{BW in kg}) \times \left[\left(\frac{\text{serum [Na}^+\text{]}}{140} \right) - 1 \right]$$

This calculated water deficit can be administered by several means. The water deficit can be provided by frequent (every 1–2 hours), small-volume feedings of water or milk over a 24-hour to 48-hour period. The amount of water fed should be minimal initially and gradually increased over the treatment period to account not only for the calculated water deficit but also for maintenance water needs and estimated water losses with diarrhea or lactation. Ideally, the water provided should be highly palatable (eg, municipal water or bottled water) to encourage consumption. For a neonate, whole milk or milk replacer formulated with palatable water sources are ideal.

Acute hypernatremia may also be treated by IV fluids such as 5% dextrose or 0.45% sodium chloride/2.5% dextrose over a 24-hour to 48-hour period.[5] These fluids lower ECF osmolarity relatively rapidly. A more conservative approach is to administer a relatively sodium-rich fluid such as isotonic saline solution (0.9% saline). After 6 to 12 hours, the IV fluid can be changed to a solution with a lower sodium concentration (see **Table 1**). If metabolic acidosis is present, administration of isotonic (1.3%) sodium bicarbonate solution or slightly hypertonic (1.4%) sodium bicarbonate solution can be administered.

Fluid Therapy for Chronic Hypernatremia

In chronic (>48 hour) hypernatremia, the potential exists for the ICF of brain cells to contain idiogenic osmoles and an increased sodium concentration. Slow correction of hypernatremia is recommended to avoid brain edema. To maximize patient safety, hypernatremia of unknown duration should be treated as chronic if the clinical history does not strongly support an acute condition.[26] The calculated water deficit is estimated in a similar manner as for acute hypernatremia; however, administration of the deficit over a period of 72 hours or more has been recommended.[21] Administration of relatively sodium-rich fluid, such as 0.9% saline, would be indicated at the onset of fluid therapy,[5] with longer (24 hour) intervals used to step down the fluid to a lower sodium solution (see **Table 1**).

Alternatively, the clinician can formulate a high-sodium crystalloid solution (HSCS) for treatment of the chronically hypernatremic animal by adding sodium (as dry salt or sodium bicarbonate, if metabolic acidosis is present) to 0.9% saline.[21,60] The goal is to create a final sodium concentration in the HSCS that is approximately 10 to 15 mEq/L less than the patient's serum sodium concentration. Dry table salt (17 mEq Na^+/g) can be added to 0.9% saline to achieve the desired sodium concentration in the HSCS. The dry salt can be aseptically placed into a syringe with the plunger removed; the plunger is then replaced and fluid drawn from the saline bag to dissolve the salt, and the solubilized salt is then injected into the bag. If metabolic acidosis is present, sodium bicarbonate (13 mEq of Na^+ and HCO_3^-/g) can be added to 0.9% saline instead of salt. Another option is to add small volumes of hypertonic saline (which has a sodium concentration of 1.2 mEq/mL) to 0.9% saline. The resulting fluid is administered at a conservative rate (1–3 mL/kg/h), and the patient's neurologic status and serum sodium concentration are monitored carefully.

Ideally, the serum sodium concentration should decline by no more than 0.3 to 1.0 mEq/L per hour, with a decline of 0.5 mEq/L/h considered a reasonable target.[56] To predict the effect of 1 L of a particular IV fluid on the patient's serum sodium concentration, the following formula can be used.[1] Sodium concentrations are in mEq/L and BW is in kg.

$$\text{Expected change in serum } [Na^+] = \frac{\text{IV fluid } [Na^+] - \text{serum } [Na^+]}{(0.6 \times BW) + 1}$$

Even with such formulas to guide therapy, redistribution of sodium in the body fluids and ongoing losses through feces or urine can impart variability to the resulting serum sodium concentration.[56]

If the patient's neurologic status allows for drinking, very small volumes of free water can be administered orally as water or milk. The exact volume to administer remains undefined, but administration of water or milk at 0.5% of BW every 2 to 4 hours seems to be a conservative rate.

If seizures develop, control can be achieved with diazepam (0.01–0.2 mg/kg IV every 30 minutes as needed) or phenobarbital (12–20 mg/kg IV slowly over 30 minutes).[25] Supplemental oxygen should be provided by nasal insufflation. Mannitol (0.25–2 g/kg of a 20% solution IV over 30–60 minutes) can be used to treat cerebral edema. Adjunct treatment with nonsteroidal antiinflammatory drugs (eg, flunixin meglumine, 1.1–2.2 mg/kg IV every 24 hours) or corticosteroids (eg, dexamethasone, 1.0–4.0 mg/kg IV) can be considered on a case-by-case basis.[25] Use of corticosteroids in NWCs may provoke hyperglycemia and complicate water balance through induction of glucose diuresis, so its use is discouraged.

Fluid Therapy for the Hyperosmolar Syndrome in Crias

In cases reported in the literature, treatment of hyperglycemia seems to be pivotal to correcting water loss in urine induced by glucose diuresis. Once glycemic control is established, the hypernatremia induced by free water loss from the ECF is corrected. Regular insulin (0.2 U/kg IV every 1–4 hours[37] or as a continuous rate infusion at 0.02 U/kg/h[35]) or ultralente insulin (0.4 U/kg SC every 24 hours)[38] should be implemented to resolve the hyperglycemia. Recently, more consistent glycemic control has been achieved in hyperglycemic NWCs by use of NPH (neutral prot-amine Hagedorn) insulin at 0.4 U/kg SC every 6 to 12 hours (S. Byers, unpublished data, 2013). Frequent (every 2–6 hours) measurement of serum glucose is recom-mended to monitor the decline in hyperglycemia; some animals may require larger doses of insulin. In addition to insulin therapy, administration of polyionic IV fluids (see **Table 1**)[34,35] is used to correct the concurrent hypernatremia. However, the exact rate of fluid administration that is safe remains undefined. Cebra[37,38] recom-mends an initial IV polyionic, sodium-containing fluid bolus equal to 2% to 4% of BW to crias (depending on degree of dehydration), with tube feeding of the dam's or goat's milk at a rate of 1% to 1.5% of BW every 2 to 3 hours to provide a source of free water to replace that lost in urine.[37] If concurrent IV fluid therapy is maintained, slow infusion of a conservative volume is recommended.[37] Moni-toring and treatment of neurologic complications are conducted as for chronic hypernatremia.

Acute Hyponatremia (<48 hours)

Acute, mild to moderate hyponatremia (serum Na^+ level = 125–135 mEq/L) is com-mon in neonatal ruminants with diarrhea.[39,61] In these cases, IV treatment with sodium-containing, isotonic fluids typically corrects the underlying hyponatremia without consequence. Similar experiences with acute, moderate hyponatremia in horses have been reported.[62,63] Isotonic (1.3%) or mildly hypertonic (1.4%)[39] solutions of sodium bicarbonate can be used with metabolic acidosis secondary to diarrhea. Hyperosmotic oral electrolyte solutions are commonly used to treat fluid and electro-lyte losses in diarrhea; restoration of eunatremia is expected over several hours if acute, mild hyponatremia exists.[64]

Severe, acute hyponatremia is considered rare in large animals, but small boluses (2.2 mL/kg) of hypertonic (7.2%) saline have been used to partially correct apparently acute, severe hyponatremia (serum Na^+ level = 99 mEq/L) in a foal.[58] Normal (0.9%) saline and isotonic (1.3%) sodium bicarbonate were subsequently used to further cor-rect the hyponatremia, along with mannitol, dimethyl sulfoxide, and corticosteroids to counter any concurrent cerebral edema and anoxia.[58] However, because of the diffi-culty in defining the duration of hyponatremia, Sterns[57] has questioned the rationale of rapid correction of severe hyponatremia in any patient. Because hyponatremia seems rare in NWCs, the magnitude of hyponatremia that is considered severe in these spe-cies has not been well defined.[65]

Chronic Hyponatremia (>48 hours)

In chronic hyponatremia, solute egress from brain cells makes the patient suscep-tible to ODS if the serum sodium concentration is increased too rapidly. As for hypernatremia, if the duration of hyponatremia cannot be accurately determined, it is most prudent to assume that the hyponatremia has existed long enough to put the patient at potential risk of ODS and treat the condition as chronic hyponatremia.

No access to salt should be provided. The amount of sodium needed to increase the serum sodium to a modestly low level (125 mEq/L in horses)[62] can be estimated using the following formula:

$$Total\ Na^+\ required\ (mEq) = (125 - serum\ [Na^+]) \times (0.6 \times BW)$$

where serum Na^+ is in mEq/L and BW is in kg.

In horses, the total sodium dose calculated according to this equation has been recommended to be delivered over a 6-hour period,[62] using a sodium-depleted fluid such as 0.45% sodium chloride/2.5% dextrose, LRS, or a fluid formulated to have a sodium concentration intermediate to these 2 standard solutions.

As for acute hyponatremia, the following formula can be used to predict the effect of 1 L of a particular IV fluid on the patient's serum sodium concentration[1]:

$$Expected\ change\ in\ serum\ [Na^+] = \frac{IV\ fluid\ [Na^+] - serum\ [Na^+]}{(0.6 \times BW) + 1}$$

where serum Na^+ is in mEq/L and BW is in kg.

The rate of correction of chronic hyponatremia has been a focus of concern in human and veterinary medicine. Based on guidelines in humans, the rate of sodium correction should not exceed 0.5 to 1.0 mEq Na^+/L/h to avoid induction of neurologic disease.[1,57] The optimal period to target for complete correction of chronic hyponatremia remains undefined, but a period of 72 hours to several (7–10) days has been proposed.[26] If neurologic signs develop during treatment, fluid therapy should be discontinued, and the serum sodium concentration measured. Diazepam or phenobarbital may be used to control seizures, and furosemide (0.5–10 mg/kg IV) may be used to lower the serum sodium concentration. If nonfatal ODS does occur, gradual resolution of neurologic signs has been reported in 1 dog receiving nonspecific supportive care.[59]

Prevention

Given the morbidity and potentially high mortality associated with severe dysnatremias, along with the expense of critical care to correct these disorders, prevention is essential in livestock medicine. Housing, shade, mist cooling systems, bedding, and ventilation should be evaluated to ensure that insensible water losses are mitigated. Camelids should be shorn appropriately. Animals at risk of overexertion (eg, males pacing the fence line of a pen of females) should be moved to a location that does not provoke this behavior. A pond, wading pool, or low sprinklers may help NWCs dissipate heat via their sparsely fibered ventrum and limbs.[52]

Animals of all ages should have ad libitum access to high-quality (pure) water; saline or high-sulfate water should be purified to optimize intake. Sources of salt should always be placed near a reliable source of palatable water. Whenever possible, locate water and salt in areas where animals seek shelter or shade. When weaning animals, it is optimal to remove the dams from the pasture or pen, leaving the weanlings in the familiar location so that the location of shade, water, and salt are known. If animals that are used to drinking from ponds or streams are moved into a corral or pen (eg, a feedlot), water should be allowed to trickle into troughs to create the familiar sound of moving water and promote more rapid recognition of water sources.

REFERENCES

1. Adrogue HJ, Madias NE. Aiding fluid prescription for the dysnatremias. Intensive Care Med 1997;23:309–16.

2. Carlson GP. Clinical chemistry tests. In: Smith BP, editor. Large animal internal medicine. 4th edition. St Louis (MO): Mosby; 2009. p. 375–97.

3. Garry F, Weiser MG, Belknap E. Clinical pathology of llamas. Vet Clin North Am Food Anim Pract 1994;10:201–9.

4. James KM, Lunn KF. An in-depth look: normal and abnormal water balance: hyponatremia and hypernatremia. Comp Cont Ed Pract Vet 2007;29:589–608.

5. Ross LA. Disorders of serum sodium concentration: diagnosis and therapy. Comp Cont Ed Pract Vet 1990;12:1277–89.

6. Guyton AC, Hall JE. The body fluid compartments: extracellular and intracellular fluids; interstitial fluid and edema. Textbook of Medical Physiology. 10th edition. Philadelphia: WB Saunders; 2000. p. 264–78.

7. Lien YH, Shapiro JI. Hyponatremia: clinical diagnosis and management. Am J Med 2007;120:653–8.

8. Bagshaw SM, Townsend DR, McDermid RC. Disorders of sodium and water balance in hospitalized patients. Can J Anaesth 2009;56:151–67.

9. Green RA. Perspectives of clinical osmometry. Vet Clin North Am 1978;8:287–99.

10. Gennari FJ. Current concepts: serum osmolality. N Engl J Med 1984;310:102–5.

11. Crowell WA, Whitlock RH, Stout RC, et al. Ethylene glycol toxicosis in cattle. Cornell Vet 1979;69:272–9.

12. Boermans HJ, Ruegg PL, Leach M. Ethylene glycol toxicosis in a pygmy goat. J Am Vet Med Assoc 1988;193:694–6.

13. Guyton AC, Hall JE. Regulation of extracellular fluid osmolarity and sodium concentration. Textbook of Medical Physiology. 10th edition. Philadelphia: WB Saunders; 2000. p. 313–28.

14. Briggs J, Singh I, Schnermann J. Disorders of sodium balance. In: Kokko J, Harvey J, Bruss M, editors. Fluid and electrolytes. 3rd edition. Philadelphia: WB Saunders; 1996. p. 3–62.

15. Guyton AC, Hall JE. Dominant role of the kidney in long-term regulation of arterial pressure and hypertension: the integrated system for volume control. Textbook of Medical Physiology. 10th edition. Philadelphia: WB Saunders; 2000. p. 195–209.

16. Guyton AC, Hall JE. The adrenocortical hormones. Textbook of Medical Physiology. 10th edition. Philadelphia: WB Saunders; 2000. p. 869–83.

17. Levin ER, Gardner DG, Samson WK. Natriuretic peptides. N Engl J Med 1998;339:321–8.

18. National Research Council. Nutrient requirements of small ruminants: sheep, goats, cervids, and New World camelids. Washington, DC: The National Academies Press; 2007. p. 183–4.

19. National Research Council. Nutrient requirements of beef cattle. Washington, DC: The National Academies Press; 2000. p. 80–2.

20. National Research Council. Nutrient requirements of dairy cattle. Washington, DC: The National Academies Press; 2001. p. 178–83.

21. Angelos SM, Smith BP, George LW, et al. Treatment of hypernatremia in an acidotic neonatal calf. J Am Vet Med Assoc 1999;214:1364–7.

22. Ollivett TL, McGuirk SM. Salt poisoning as a cause of morbidity and mortality in neonatal dairy calves. J Vet Intern Med 2013;27:592–5.

23. Adrogue HJ, Madias NE. Hyponatremia. N Engl J Med 2000;342:1581–9.

24. Gullans SR, Verbalis JG. Control of brain volume during hyperosmolar and hypoosmolar conditions. Annu Rev Med 1993;44:289–301.

25. Smith MO, George LW. Diseases of the nervous system. In: Smith BP, editor. Large animal internal medicine. 4th edition. St Louis (MO): Mosby; 2009. p. 972–1111.

26. Angelos SM, Van Metre DC. Treatment of sodium balance disorders. Vet Clin North Am Food Anim Pract 1999;15:587–607.

27. Utter MF. Mechanism of inhibition of anaerobic glycolysis of brain by sodium ions. J Biol Chem 1950;185:499–517.

28. Pringle JK, Berthiaume LM. Hypernatremia in calves. J Vet Intern Med 1988;2: 66–70.

29. Abutarbush SM, Petrie L. Treatment of hypernatremia in neonatal calves with diarrhea. Can Vet J 2007;48:184–7.

30. Constable PD. Fluid and electrolyte therapy in ruminants. Vet Clin North Am Food Anim Pract 2003;19:557–97.

31. Roussel AJ, Cohen ND, Holland PS, et al. Alterations in acid-base balance and serum electrolyte concentrations in cattle: 632 cases (1984-1994). J Am Vet Med Assoc 1998;212:1769–75.

32. Arieff AI. Effects of water, acid-base, and electrolyte disorders on the central nervous system. In: Arieff AI, DeFronzio RA, editors. Fluid, electrolyte, and acid-base disorders. New York: Churchill Livingstone; 1985. p. 969–1040.

33. Lein YH, Shapiro JI, Chan L. Effects of hypernatremia on organic brain osmoles. J Clin Invest 1990;85:1427–35.

34. Cebra CK. Hyperglycemia, hypernatremia, and hyperosmolarity in 6 neonatal llamas and alpacas. J Am Vet Med Assoc 2000;217:1701–4.

35. Buchheit TM, Sommardahl CS, Frank N, et al. Use of a constant rate infusion of insulin for the treatment of hyperglycemic, hypernatremic, hyperosmolar syndrome in an alpaca cria. J Am Vet Med Assoc 2010;236:566.

36. Kozikowski TA, Magdesian KG, Puschner B. Oleander intoxication in New World camelids: 12 cases (1995–2006). J Am Vet Med Assoc 2009;235:305–10.

37. Cebra CK. Disorders of carbohydrate or lipid metabolism in camelids. Vet Clin North Am Food Anim Pract 2009;25:339–52.

38. Cebra C. Practical fluid therapy. In Large Animal Proceedings, North American Veterinary Conference. Florida; 2006; p. 273–74.

39. Muller KR, Gentile A, Klee W, et al. Importance of the effective strong ion difference of an intravenous solution in the treatment of diarrheic calves with naturally acquired academia and strong ion (metabolic) acidosis. J Vet Intern Med 2012; 26:674–83.

40. Massip A. Hematocrit, biochemical and plasma cortisol changes associated with diarrhea in the calf. Br Vet J 1979;135:600–5.

41. Chamorro MF, Passler T, Joiner K, et al. Acute renal failure in 2 adult llamas after exposure to oak trees (*Quercus* spp.). Can Vet J 2013;54:61–4.

42. Hutchison JM, Belknap EB, Williams RJ. Acute renal failure in the llama (*Lama glama*). Cornell Vet 1993;83:39–46.

43. Mechor GD, Cebra CK. Renal failure in a calf secondary to chronic enteritis. Cornell Vet 1993;83:325–31.

44. Brobst DF, Parish SM, Trobeck RL, et al. Azotemia in cattle. J Am Vet Med Assoc 1978;173:481–5.

45. Garry F, Chew DJ, Hoffsis GF. Urinary indices of renal function in sheep with induced aminoglycoside nephrotoxicosis. Am J Vet Res 1990;51:420–7.

46. Hinchcliff KW, Shaftoe S, Dubielzig RR. Gentamicin-induced nephrotoxicosis in a cow. J Am Vet Med Assoc 1988;192:923–5.

47. Spier SJ, Smith BP, Seawright AA, et al. Oak toxicosis in cattle: clinical and pathological findings. J Am Vet Med Assoc 1987;191:958–64.

48. Divers TJ, Crowell WA, Duncan JR, et al. Acute renal disorders in cattle: a retrospective study of 22 cases. J Am Vet Med Assoc 1982;181:694–9.

49. Sockett DC, Knight AP, Fettman MJ, et al. Metabolic changes due to experimentally induced rupture of the bovine urinary bladder. Cornell Vet 1986;76: 198–212.

50. von Duvillard SP, Braun WA, Markofski M, et al. Fluids and hydration in prolonged endurance performance. Nutrition 2004;20:651–6.

51. Hausfater P, Mégarbane B, Fabricatore L, et al. Serum sodium abnormalities during nonexertional heatstroke: incidence and prognostic values. Am J Emerg Med 2012;30:741–8.

52. Middleton JR, Parish SM. Heat stress in a llama (Lama glama): a case report and review of the syndrome. J Camel Pract Res 1999;6:265–9.

53. Tennant B, Harrold D, Reina-Guerra M. Hypoglycemia in neonatal calves associated with diarrhea. Cornell Vet 1968;58:136–46.

54. Trefz FM, Lorch A, Feist M, et al. The prevalence and clinical relevance of hyperkalemia in calves with neonatal diarrhea. Vet J 2013;195:350–6.

55. Cluitmans FH, Meinders AE. Management of severe hyponatremia: rapid or slow correction? Am J Med 1990;88:161–6.

56. Wong DM, Sponseller BT, Brockus C, et al. Neurologic deficits associated with severe hyponatremia in 2 foals. J Vet Emerg Crit Care 2007;17:275–85.

57. Sterns RH. The treatment of hyponatremia: first do no harm [editorial]. Am J Med 1990;88:557–60.

58. Lakritz J, Madigan J, Carlson GP. Hypovolemic hyponatremia and signs of neurologic disease associated with diarrhea in a foal. J Am Vet Med Assoc 1992;200:1114–6.

59. O'Brien DP, Kroll RA, Johnson GC, et al. Myelinolysis after correction of hyponatremia in two dogs. J Vet Intern Med 1994;8:40–8.

60. Banks P, Roussel AJ, Mealey RH. High-sodium crystalloid solution for treatment of hypernatremia in a Vietnamese pot-bellied pig. J Am Vet Med Assoc 1996; 209:1268–70.

61. Tennant B, Harrold D, Reina-Guerra M. Physiologic and metabolic factors in the pathogenesis of neonatal enteric infections in calves. J Am Vet Med Assoc 1972;161:993–1007.

62. Holbrook TC. Slow versus rapid correction of hyponatremia in horses. Comp Cont Ed Pract Vet 1993;15:1096–9.

63. Johnson PJ. Electrolyte and acid-base disorders in the horse. Vet Clin North Am Equine Pract 1995;111:491–514.

64. Jones R, Philips RW, Cleek JL. Hyperosmotic oral replacement fluid for diarrheic calves. J Am Vet Med Assoc 1984;184:1501–5.

65. Cebra C. Diarrhea in llama and alpaca crias. In: Smith RA, editor. Proceedings of the Fortieth Annual Conference. Vancouver (Canada): American Association of Bovine Practitioners; 2007. p. 170–3.

Hypokalemia Syndrome in Cattle

Nicolas Sattler[a], Gilles Fecteau[b,*]

KEYWORDS

- Bovine • Hypokalemia • Recumbency • Electrolytes • Anorexia • Potassium

KEY POINTS

- Risk factors for hypokalemia syndrome include the early lactation period, anorexia, and repeated administration of isoflupredone.
- Treatment includes basic supportive care for recumbent animals and aggressive potassium replacement therapy.
- Prognosis is guarded for recumbent cattle and worsens if hypokalemic myopathy or complications of recumbency occur.

INTRODUCTION

Total body potassium depletion leads to muscle weakness and may or may not be associated with low plasma potassium concentration (hypokalemia). More often, hypokalemia is observed on a serum biochemistry profile in animals without potassium depletion (potassium redistribution). The clinical significance of hypokalemia cannot be ascertained without considering the other electrolytes as well as the acid-base status. Moreover, the physical examination and complete history dictate whether intervention is necessary.

NORMAL POTASSIUM BALANCE

Potassium is mostly intracellular. Serum potassium concentration is a poor indicator of the potassium status of the animal. Determination of intracellular potassium concentration in erythrocytes or muscle cells is a more accurate way to assess potassium depletion, but with current technology it is not clinically feasible in most cases.[1,2]

The concentration of potassium in plasma depends on external potassium balance and internal potassium balance. External potassium balance refers to potassium

The authors have nothing to disclose.

[a] Service Vétérinaire Saint-Vallier, 400 montée de la station, Saint-Vallier, Québec, G0R3J0 Canada; [b] Clinical Sciences Department, Faculté de Médecine Vétérinaire, Université de Montréal, Saint-Hyacinthe, Québec J2S 7C6, Canada

* Corresponding author.

E-mail address: gilles.fecteau@umontreal.ca

Vet Clin Food Anim 30 (2014) 351–357

http://dx.doi.org/10.1016/j.cvfa.2014.04.004

vetfood.theclinics.com

intake and absorption from the gastrointestinal (GI) tract, and potassium excretion by the kidneys. The primary source of potassium is the forage portion of the normal ruminant diet. An animal with a normal appetite usually has a normal serum potassium concentration. Almost all ingested potassium (more than 300 g per day for a 600-kg cow) is absorbed and reaches the intracellular fluid compartment. Because they have a forage-based diet, lactating dairy cows may eat more than 10 times their daily potassium requirement. For this reason, cattle have renal excretory mechanisms that are well developed to eliminate the excess potassium load from the body. When intake is interrupted, the excretory mechanisms may not respond rapidly enough to avoid potassium depletion. Cows with partial and/or total anorexia frequently have moderate hypokalemia. This hypokalemia is not coupled with clinical signs of weakness. Other abnormalities such as diarrhea, third space loss, and alkalosis can exacerbate potassium loss from the intracellular and extracellular fluid compartments.

Some corticosteroids with mineralocorticoid effects are known to lead to hypokalemia (eg, isoflupredone acetate) by increasing potassium excretion in the kidneys. Diuretic drugs (eg, furosemide) may also contribute to renal potassium loss. Following relief of a urinary obstruction, a diuretic phase occurs and may lead to significant potassium loss.

Internal potassium balance refers to the distribution of potassium between the intracellular fluid (ICF) compartment and extracellular fluid (ECF) compartment. Acid-base balance has a significant effect on the distribution of potassium between these compartments, with acidosis causing the movement of potassium from the ICF to the ECF and resulting in hyperkalemia, and alkalosis causing potassium movement in the other direction resulting in hypokalemia. Insulin also facilitates the movement of potassium from the ECF to the ICF. Therefore, the administration of dextrose or insulin may result in hypokalemia or an amelioration of hyperkalemia if it exists.

THE CLINICAL SYNDROME
Introduction

Hypokalemia syndrome has been reported.[3–6] Lactating dairy cows as well as younger animals may develop the disease. At present, except for animals treated with repeated isoflupredone acetate administrations, the exact determinants causing hypokalemia syndrome remain uncertain.

Risk Factors

Lactating dairy cows less than 60 days in milk seem to be at greatest risk. Systemic illness causing anorexia of several days' duration is a risk factor.[4] Repeated systemic or intramammary administration of isoflupredone acetate can cause the syndrome. The mineralocorticoid activity of isoflupredone acetate disturbs both the internal and external potassium balance.[7] Repeated doses can reduce serum potassium concentration by 70%.[8] Food-restricted dairy cattle receiving repeated doses of isoflupredone acetate developed the syndrome in an experimental model.[9] Following the label directions concerning dose and duration seems to be important. Although it is a less potent mineralocorticoid, use of dexamethasone was also reported as a potential cause in some cases.[4,6]

Multiple treatments of dextrose and insulin are also reported to be associated with the syndrome.[3–6] In young animals, the repeated administration of isoflupredone acetate to treat pneumonia and intravenous (IV) fluid administration have been reported to initiate the syndrome.[4]

Clinical Signs

In most cases, a primary disease was diagnosed and treated by either the owner or a veterinarian before the generalized weakness or recumbency developed. The identification of the concomitant disease is essential and should not be overlooked because it influences the recovery and prognosis. Some patients are presented with an obscure GI problem: anorexia, little to no feces, reluctance to move, and rapid return to recumbency after stimulation to get up, mimicking colic. In most cases, the animal rapidly becomes incapable of getting up and severe paresis develops. This constellation of signs creates some confusion in the management of the case; specifically, whether surgery is indicated.

After the initial phase of stiffness and tendency to lie down, most animals develop the following clinical signs:

- Severe apparent depression (generalized weakness with little resistance to any manipulations)
- Lack of tone of most muscle groups (tail tone to tongue tone are reduced)
- Tachycardia
- Abnormal neck posture (S-shaped neck) (**Fig. 1**)
- Recumbency
- GI stasis (forestomach and intestine) so no ruminal motility and little if any feces

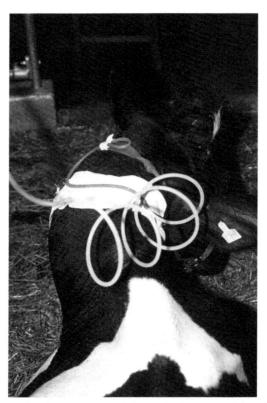

Fig. 1. Typical (or classic) S-shape position of the neck of a cow with hypokalemia. The neck muscle tone is so weak that the head cannot be held straight.

In our experience, 2 types of recumbent animals may be observed. Some are weak to the point of being unable to rise but do not have severe generalized rhabdomyolysis, whereas others have severe rhabdomyolysis even in the non–weight-bearing muscle groups. The patients with severe rhabdomyolysis recuperate slower, even after the serum potassium value returns to normal. The increase in creatine kinase and aspartate aminotransferase are more pronounced in the second group.

The generalized weakness often prevents the animal from reaching for food or water, and it is common to observe a cow eating her grain if her head is placed in the feed bucket. Perhaps an apparent lack of appetite can be explained by the inability to reach the feed rather than anorexia. The position of the head is worth describing in more detail. There is a complete inability to keep the head in a straight position. The neck is carried in an S-shaped posture. Lack of muscle tone allows easy movement of the head. Sometimes it is possible to position the head and neck in their normal straight position, but inevitably the head eventually falls to one side or the other. The first few cases of hypokalemia syndrome diagnosed by the authors were initially suspected to have cervical subluxation because of this awkward positioning of the neck. This condition may be observed in the standing animal immediately before recumbency occurs or in the recumbent patient. Cardiac dysrhythmias may also be noted (ventricular tachycardia, accelerated escape ventricular rhythm, or atrial fibrillation).[4]

Pathophysiology

Because most of the total body potassium is intracellular,[10] plasma concentration is not as important as the gradient between the potassium concentrations of the ICF and ECF compartments, which is the determinant of the resting cellular membrane potential and plays a role in the formation and transmission of action potentials.[11] This gradient explains why animals may be observed with weakness in the absence of severe rhabdomyolysis. However, structural damage associated with potassium depletion has also been reported in cattle.[3–5,12] This structural damage most likely occurs in the group of patients observed with severe rhabdomyolysis. As far as the authors know and according to other investigators, there is no clear explanation for the distribution of animals into one category or the other.[3,4]

The changes in cardiac electrical activity associated with hypokalemia could be explained by one or more of the following phenomena: hyperpolarization of the cardiac cell resulting in spontaneous automatic activity, slow conduction caused by the increased difference between resting membrane potential and threshold potential, increased action potential duration as a result of slow repolarization, depressed fast responses because of higher membrane potential when a slow repolarizing cell is stimulated, slow responses in fibers normally showing fast responses, and conduction block.[13] In addition to electrical abnormalities, if muscle cell necrosis occurs, cardiac dysrhythmia could become even more likely. However, muscle lesions compatible with hypokalemic myopathy (muscular necrosis) have not been consistently documented in the reported hypokalemia syndrome of cattle.[3–6]

Differential Diagnosis

In the early stages of the condition, hypokalemia syndrome could be confused with GI problems such as acute abdomen: intestinal ileus and intussusception or musculoskeletal/neurologic problems such as cervical trauma, luxations, osteomyelitis or neoplasia, vertebral malformations, fractures, and torticollis. A complete history and thorough physical examination help rule out the other possibilities mentioned earlier. Other conditions to rule out when the animal is presented recumbent are hypocalcemia, botulism, and tick paralysis. It is important to consider hypokalemia syndrome as a differential diagnosis in recumbent postpartum cows because administration of calcium solution intravenously to normocalcemic cows carries a substantial risk.

Clinical Pathology and Ancillary Tests

Serum biochemistry profile is helpful in the management of hypokalemic cattle. However, there is no consensus on the lower threshold for potassium below which the diagnosis is confirmed. The lower threshold limit is usually stated to be 2.2 to 2.5 mmol/L. The degree of increase of creatine phosphokinase and other muscle enzymes suggests whether the muscle damage is related to the primary problem (hypokalemia) or to secondary (recumbency-associated) muscle damage. Concomitant acid-base derangements vary from severe metabolic hypochloremic alkalosis to metabolic acidosis in severe advanced cases.[3] Hypophosphatemia has been observed in 25% to 40% of cases but the significance of this finding remains to be shown.[3–5]

Lumbar muscle biopsy (between L2 and L5) on a living patient or sampling during postmortem examination helps to differentiate primary hypokalemic myopathy from secondary myopathy caused by recumbency.

Fractional urinary excretion of potassium (FE$_k$) has been used to provide insight into the pathophysiology of hypokalemia syndrome. In one study, FE$_k$ remained in the normal to high range despite a documented severe hypokalemia 12 to 24 hours before clinical signs appeared. FE$_k$ from 55% to 128% have been reported in 5 hypokalemia cases.[5] The normal range of FE$_k$ for early lactating cattle has been reported to be 26.9% to 120%.[14]

A method of determining both the internal and external potassium balances simultaneously in dairy cows has been presented.[3]

Treatment

Nonspecific treatment

Any concomitant or preexisting problems should be addressed appropriately. Good nursing care appropriate for any down cow should be in place and emphasized. Of particular importance is keeping feed and water easily accessible to the cow at all times. Dairy cows should be milked regularly and turned from one side to the other. Any device helping the animal to get up is useful, but the timing is important. Premature attempts may aggravate or cause a musculoskeletal problem because weak animals are prone to injury (lack of muscle tone). Use of a flotation tank (Aquacow Rise System) is of great value once the serum potassium concentration has returned to the normal range.

Specific treatment

If serious complications arise during the animal's recumbency, even if normal potassium status is restored, the complicating problem may result in the death of the animal. Good nursing care is critical to the recovery of hypokalemic patients. Specific treatment is intended to address potassium depletion. Potassium chloride supplementation administered orally is the preferred method. The optimal total amount to administer daily remains to be defined, but the authors have used 60 to 100 g/100 kg of body weight per day. However, most investigators recommend a lower dose (250 g per cow per day). When IV potassium chloride is administered, the rate should not exceed 0.5 mEq of K$^+$/kg/h. Serum potassium should be monitored daily to allow adjustment of the treatment regimen. Treatment is usually necessary for 3 to 5 days.[3–5] It is probably safe to continue some supplementation until the appetite has returned to 100%.

Prevention

Prevention is oriented toward supplementation of animals considered to be at risk. Dairy cattle that are chronically anorectic and treated with isoflupredone acetate and/or IV dextrose and insulin should received oral potassium supplementation. The optimal dosage regimen to administer to a normal patient considered at risk is empiric, but 100 g twice a day seems safe.

Prognosis

In 3 reports, the survival rates were 2 of 8,[3] 7 of 17,[5] and 11 of 14.[4] The survival rate in retrospective studies is inconsistent because so many variables accounted for death and/or euthanasia (duration of recumbency, severity of concomitant disease, presence of hypokalemic myopathy, and treatments received, as well as cost of treatment in a particular hospital).[1] Prevention of any complications associated with recumbency is probably a major determinant in the outcome. The complexity of the disease and the duration of the recovery phase warrant a guarded prognosis at best. The availability of a flotation tank seems to be a significant positive prognostic factor.[3–5]

UNANSWERED QUESTIONS

A few important questions remain unanswered. The precise relationship between the perturbations of internal versus external potassium balance in affected cattle is not clear. The precipitating factor for some cattle to develop the severe rhabdomyolysis is still not understood. The impact of excessive nutritional potassium on kidney homeostasis should be investigated further. The optimal treatment regimen is also still to be proved in a clinical trial.

REFERENCES

1. Johnson PJ, Goetz TE, Foreman JH, et al. Effect of whole-body potassium depletion on plasma, erythrocyte, and middle gluteal muscle potassium concentration of healthy, adult horses. Am J Vet Res 1991;52:1676–83.
2. Sattler N, Fecteau G, Couture Y, et al. Évaluation des équilibres potassiques chez la vache laitière et étude de ses variations journalières et selon le stade de production. Can Vet J 2001;42:107–15.
3. Sielman ES, Sweeney RW, Whitlock RH, et al. Hypokalemia syndrome in dairy cows: 10 cases (1992–1996). J Am Vet Med Assoc 1997;210:240–3.
4. Sattler N, Fecteau G, Girard C, et al. Description of 14 cases of bovine hypokalaemia syndrome. Vet Rec 1998;143:503–7.
5. Peek SF, Divers TJ, Guard C, et al. Hypokalemia, muscle weakness and recumbency in dairy cattle. Vet Ther 2000;1:235–44.
6. Johns IC, Whitlock RH, Sweeney RW. Hypokalaemia as a cause of recumbency in an adult dairy cow. Aust Vet J 2004;82:413–6.
7. Vita G, Bartolone S, Santoro M, et al. Hypokalemic myopathy in pseudohyperaldosteronism induced by fluoroprednisolone-containing nasal spray. Clin Neuropathol 1987;6:80–5.
8. Neff AW, Connor AD, Bryan HS. Studies on 9α-fluoroprednisolone acetate, a new synthetic corticosteroid for the treatment of bovine ketosis. J Dairy Sci 1960;43:553–62.

9. Sattler N, Fecteau G, Pare J. Experimental reproduction of the bovine hypokalemia syndrome [abstract]. J Vet Intern Med 2002;16:337.
10. Guyton AC, Hall JE. Transport of ions and molecules through the cell membrane. In: Guyton AC, Hall JE, editors. Textbook of medical physiology. 9th edition. Philadelphia: WB Saunders; 1996. p. 43–55.
11. Guyton AC, Hall JE. Membrane potentials and action potentials. In: Guyton AC, Hall JE, editors. Textbook of medical physiology. 9th edition. Philadelphia: WB Saunders; 1996. p. 57–72.
12. Lindeman RD. Hypokalemia: causes, consequences and correction. Am J Med Sci 1976;272:5–17.
13. Commerford PJ, Lloyd EA. Arrhythmias in patients with drug toxicity, electrolyte and endocrine disturbances. Med Clin North Am 1984;68:1051–78.
14. Fleming SA, Hunt EL, Brownie C, et al. Fractional excretion of electrolytes in lactating dairy cows. Am J Vet Res 1992;53:222–4.

Calcium and Magnesium Disorders

Jesse P. Goff, DVM, PhD

KEYWORDS

- Milk fever • DCAD • Hypomagnesemia • Hypocalcemia • Parathyroid hormone

KEY POINTS

- Hypocalcemia is a clinical disorder that can be life threatening to the cow (milk fever) and predisposes the animal to various other metabolic and infectious disorders.
- Calcium homeostasis is mediated primarily by parathyroid hormone, which stimulates bone calcium resorption and renal calcium reabsorption.
- Parathyroid hormone stimulates the production of 1,25-dihydroxyvitamin D to enhance diet calcium absorption.
- High dietary cation-anion difference interferes with tissue sensitivity to parathyroid hormone.
- Hypomagnesemia reduces tissue response to parathyroid hormone.

IMPACT OF HYPOCALCEMIA ON COW HEALTH

Total blood calcium (Ca) concentration in the adult cow is maintained between 8.5 and 10.0 mg/dL (2.1 and 2.5 mmol/L). Nearly all cows will experience some degree of hypocalcemia at the onset of lactation; however, the severity and duration of the hypocalcemia experienced depends on the integrity of the cow's Ca homeostasis mechanisms. Typically, the nadir in blood Ca concentration occurs 12 to 24 hours after calving. Surveys in the United States suggest around 5% of cows will develop milk fever each year[1]; the incidence of subclinical hypocalcemia (blood Ca values between 5.5 and 8.0 mg/dL [1.38–2.0 mmol/L] during the periparturient period) is around 50% in older cows.[2] Cows with subclinical hypocalcemia mobilize more body fat resulting in higher blood nonesterified fatty acid concentrations, increasing the risk for ketosis and displaced abomasum. Hypocalcemia reduces rumen and abomasal motility, further increasing the risk of abomasal displacement. Hypocalcemia also

Author Disclosures: Before joining the faculty at Iowa State University, J.P. Goff was Director of Research at West Central Farmer's Cooperative. In this capacity, he developed anion supplements for prevention of hypocalcemia in cows and continues to consult for this company. J.P. Goff also holds a patent using calcium propionate paste to prevent hypocalcemia.
Department of Biomedical Sciences, College of Veterinary Medicine, Iowa State University, 2048 Vet Med, Ames, IA 50011, USA
E-mail address: jpgoff@iastate.edu

Vet Clin Food Anim 30 (2014) 359–381
http://dx.doi.org/10.1016/j.cvfa.2014.04.003
0749-0720/14/$ – see front matter © 2014 Elsevier Inc. All rights reserved.

reduces the contraction of the teat sphincter muscle responsible for closure of the teat orifice after milking, thus, increasing the risk of mastitis. Hypocalcemia is accompanied by reductions in intracellular endoplasmic reticulum and mitochondria stores of Ca in blood mononuclear cells. Low intracellular stores of Ca impair the immune cell response by reducing the release of the second messenger Ca into the cytosol from intracellular stores in response to cytokines, antigens or other activating stimulus.[3] Martinez and colleagues[4] found that subclinical hypocalcemia impaired many aspects of neutrophil function, and cows with subclinical hypocalcemia had higher blood β-hydroxybutyrate concentrations than normocalcemic cows. They also concluded the relative risk of developing metritis increased by 22% for every 1 mg/dL decrease in serum Ca less than 8.59 mg/dL. Subclinical hypocalcemia increases the risk for fatty liver development and reduces fertility of the cow.[5] Milk fever and subclinical milk fever should be considered gateway diseases that greatly reduce the chance for full productivity of a cow in the ensuing lactation.

CA HOMEOSTASIS
Ca Pools Within the Body

Blood Ca in the adult cow is maintained between 8.5 and 10.0 mg/dL (2.1–2.5 mmol/L). About 50% of the Ca is bound to proteins such as albumin, and 42% to 48% of the Ca exists in the ionized form. The ionized Ca concentration is the biologically active portion of the Ca in blood. Under acidic conditions, the ionized portion of Ca in the blood is closer to 48%; under alkaline conditions, it is closer to 42% ionized. The final 3% to 7% of Ca in blood is bound to soluble anions, such as citrate, phosphate, bicarbonate, and sulfate. If total serum proteins are greatly reduced (hypoalbuminemia), it is possible to have low total Ca in the blood and relatively normal levels of ionized Ca in the blood. Serum albumin does decline slightly at calving; but this is not a major concern in periparturient cows, and this author thinks there is little to be gained clinically by adjusting blood Ca concentration for albumin content. Recent advances in ion electrode design are making cowside ionized Ca determinations practical, though total Ca concentration determinations are as useful clinically.

There are 3.0 to 3.5 g of Ca in the plasma pool and another 8 to 9 g of Ca in all the extracellular fluids (outside of bone) of a 600-kg cow (**Fig. 1**). Between 7.8 and 8.5 kg of Ca is contained within the skeleton. Less than 1 g of Ca is stored inside of all the cells of the body. Dairy cows producing colostrum (containing 1.7–2.3 g of Ca per kilogram) or milk (containing 1.1 g of Ca per kilogram) withdraw 20 to 30 g of Ca from these pools each day in the first days of lactation. In many cows, the demand for Ca increases dramatically even before calving, as Ca leaves blood and is sequestered within the mammary gland during colostrum formation. If the cow is to avoid severe or prolonged hypocalcemia at the onset of lactation, she must replace the extracellular Ca that is used to produce milk.

Role of Parathyroid Hormone

Ca homeostasis is primarily controlled by the parathyroid glands, which are exquisitely sensitive to a decline in blood Ca concentration and respond to hypocalcemia by secreting parathyroid hormone (PTH). The parathyroid cells can determine the extracellular ionized Ca concentration using Ca sensing receptor molecules, located on the surface of parathyroid cells, which have the ability to bind ionized Ca in the millimolar range. Whenever ionized Ca in the extracellular fluid decreases below the concentration needed to keep the Ca sensing receptors fully occupied, PTH is secreted in large amounts.[6] PTH is an 84 amino acid peptide that binds to receptors located on the

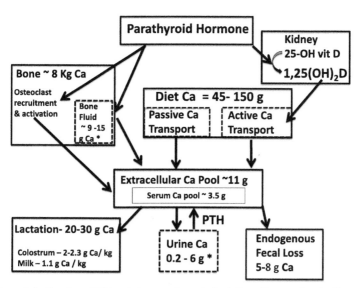

Fig. 1. Ca metabolism in a 600-kg dairy cow in early lactation. Bone osteoclastic and osteo-cytic resorption mechanisms are directly controlled by parathyroid hormone (PTH). PTH action on the kidney can increase reabsorption of Ca from glomerular filtrate and increase synthesis of 1,25-dihydroxyvitamin D (1,25[OH]$_2$D). The 1,25(OH)$_2$D can stimulate intestinal transcellular active transport of dietary Ca. In addition, some portion of dietary Ca is absorbed passively by a paracellular route driven by the concentration of ionized Ca over the tight junctions between intestinal epithelial cells. * Signifies that under acidotic conditions, the size of the bone fluid pool and the urinary Ca loss are approximated by the higher number listed in these pools. Under alkaline conditions, the size of these pools is best approximated by the lower number.

surface of its target tissues. The primary target cells are bone osteoblasts and osteo-cytes as well as renal tubular epithelial cells. The PTH receptor is a transmembrane protein with one portion extending out from the target cell into the extracellular fluid that binds PTH specifically. There is also an intracellular portion of the receptor molecule extending into the interior of the cell. PTH receptors are G-protein coupled receptors. The intracellular portion is linked to G proteins, with α, β, and γ units. The G-α (sometimes referred to as *G-stimulatory*) protein is normally in an inactive state and has a guanosine diphosphate (GDP) molecule attached to it. When PTH binds to the PTH receptor, the receptor changes its tertiary structure. Coincident with the change in shape of the PTH receptor, the G-α protein changes shape and exchanges the GDP it carries for an Mg^{++}guanosine triphosphate (Mg^{++}GTP). Binding Mg^{++} ATP further changes the conformation of the G-α protein causing it to dissociate from the PTH receptor. It then forms a complex with adenylyl cyclase located within the adjacent cell membrane. The G-α/adenylyl cyclase complex is able to convert Mg^{++} adenosine triphosphate (Mg^{++}ATP) to cyclic adenosine monophosphate (cyclic AMP).[7] The cyclic AMP serves as a second messenger to stimulate protein kinases and other pathways within each type of target cell that will help restore extracellular Ca back to normal levels (**Fig. 2A**).

Renal Ca Reabsorption

PTH has 3 major Ca elevating actions (see **Fig. 1**). Its first action is to enhance renal reabsorption of Ca from proximal renal tubular fluids. In cows fed typical diets high

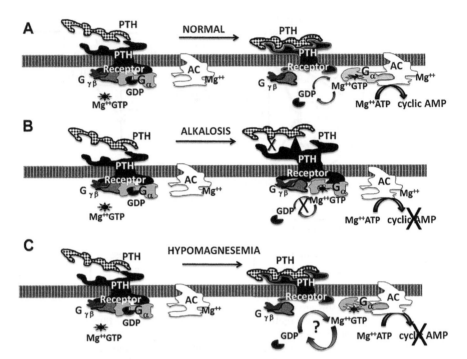

Fig. 2. Action of PTH at the cell membrane level. (*A*) PTH secreted in response to hypocalce-mia binds the PTH receptor on bone and kidney cells in a tight lock and key fit. This changes the conformation of the PTH receptor causing the G-α protein attached to its intracellular section to exchange a GDP molecule for a magnesium (Mg) GTP molecule. The G-α protein now migrates away from the PTH receptor and becomes bound to adenylyl cyclase (AC). This process activates the adenylyl cyclase, which converts Mg-ATP to cyclic AMP. The cyclic AMP then activates kinases and other enzymes to initiate processes that will return blood Ca to normal levels. (*B*) Diets high in dietary cation-anion difference induce a metabolic alkalosis, which changes the tertiary structure of the extracellular portion of the PTH receptor so it no longer binds PTH with high affinity, interfering with Ca homeostasis. (*C*) Hypomagnesemia leads to decreased intracellular Mg. The adenylyl cyclase enzyme requires Mg as a cofactor; under hypomagnesemic conditions, it cannot be fully activated. If intracellular Mg-GTP and Mg-ATP concentrations decrease, it may limit the ability of Mg-GTP to activate the G-α pro-tein and limit Mg-ATP substrate needed for production of cyclic AMP.

in dietary cation-anion difference (DCAD), urine Ca excretion is less than 0.5 g of Ca per day. If the perturbation in blood Ca is small, reducing the urinary Ca loss may be all that is required to restore blood Ca concentration to normal levels. Unfortu-nately, at the onset of lactation, the dairy cow is losing 20 to 30 g of Ca to colostrum and early milk production each day. She must use mechanisms beyond simply reducing urine Ca to remain normocalcemic. To prevent hypocalcemia, she must with-draw Ca from bone and increase the efficiency of absorption of dietary Ca.

Osteoclastic Bone Ca Resorption

Mobilizing Ca stored in bone represents a way to bring large amounts of Ca into the blood to combat hypocalcemia. Ca exists in bone in 2 forms that can contribute to Ca homeostasis. The bulk (>99%) of Ca in the skeleton is found within hydroxyapatite crystals bound to the collagen matrix. Hydroxyapatite has the general formula of 10 Ca^{+2}: 6 Phosphate (PO_4^{-3}): 2 hydroxyl anions (OH^-). Ca within these bone crystals can only be mobilized by osteoclasts, which secrete enzymes and acid to digest the collagen matrix. This action liberates the Ca and PO_4^{-2} from the crystals for return to the blood. Osteoclasts, which are related to macrophages and monocytes, do not have PTH receptors. PTH receptors are found on the osteoblasts that line all bone surfaces. The osteoblasts respond to PTH by secreting factors such as the receptor activator of nuclear factor $\kappa\beta$ ligand and macrophage colony-stimulating factor (M-CSF).[8] These cytokine factors cause preexisting osteoclasts to begin to resorb bone collagen to release Ca and cause osteoclast progenitor cells to differentiate and become new osteoclasts. It generally takes several days for osteoclastic bone resorption to become fully active.[9]

Osteocytic Osteolysis of Bone Ca

A much smaller, but very critical, amount of Ca is in the solution within the lacunae surrounding each osteocyte and the canaliculi system connecting osteocytes within the bone. This bone fluid compartment is completely lined by osteocytes and osteocyte processes and is separate from, but in equilibrium with, extracellular fluids. This Ca is readily mobilized, and the osteocytes lining this compartment respond within minutes to PTH by pumping bone fluid Ca into the extracellular fluid.[10] The amount of Ca in the bone fluid compartment is about 9 g Ca when the cow is in a state of metabolic alkalosis and increases to about 15 g Ca when the cow is in an acidotic state.

Dietary Ca Absorption

Ultimately, diet Ca must be used efficiently if the cow is to avoid hypocalcemia. Ca, like all minerals, must be in solution if it is to cross the intestinal tract and enter the blood. Fortunately, the acids of the abomasum permit much of the inorganic dietary Ca to become solubilized. Unfortunately, much of the Ca provided by forages is bound to organic materials, such as oxalate and lignin, and is unavailable to the cow.[11,12] Soluble dietary Ca can cross the foregut and gastrointestinal epithelium by 2 mechanisms.

Vitamin D–Dependent Transcellular-Intestinal Absorption

The first mechanism involves the active transport of Ca across intestinal epithelial cells, primarily in the duodenum and jejunum, by a process that depends on the stimulation of the epithelial cells by the hormonal form of vitamin D, 1,25-dihydroxyvitamin D (1,25$[OH]_2$D). Vitamin D, synthesized in the skin of the cow following irradiation by the ultraviolet B rays of the sun or supplied in the diet, is simply a precursor for the hormone, 1,25$(OH)_2$D. The first step in production of the hormone is for the vitamin D to enter the circulation and be extracted from the blood by the liver. Here the vitamin D is hydroxylated at carbon number 25 to form 25-OH vitamin D, which is released to the circulation. This form is the major form of vitamin D found in blood, and serum levels of 25-OH vitamin D are used to assess vitamin D status. The 25-OH vitamin D then travels to the kidney. If the kidney has been properly stimulated by PTH, the 25-OH vitamin D is converted to 1,25$(OH)_2$D by the 1α-hydroxylase enzyme. The hormone 1,25$(OH)_2$D is secreted by the kidney into the blood and travels to the intestine. The hormone 1,25$(OH)_2$D is a steroid hormone that diffuses into the target cells and interacts with its receptor, the vitamin D receptor (VDR), located within the cell nucleus. VDR is found in virtually all epithelial cells of the gastrointestinal tract, where it initiates transcription and translation of genes necessary for the active transport of diet Ca across the epithelial cells.

The first obstacle to transcellular Ca transport is moving the Ca across the apical membrane of the cells. Because intracellular ionized Ca concentrations are extremely low, virtually all diets contain enough Ca to ensure the Ca concentration in the lumen of the gut exceeds the Ca concentration inside the epithelial cells lining the intestinal tract. This concentration difference creates an electrochemical gradient that would drive Ca across the apical membrane if the membrane were freely permeable to Ca. However, the cell membrane is not freely permeable to Ca. One function of $1,25(OH)_2D$ is to stimulate the production of apical membrane Ca channel proteins, such as the transient receptor potential cation channel, subfamily V protein (TRPV-6). Opening of the TRPV-6 channel allows Ca to reach the cytosol. Now the Ca becomes bound to a second vitamin D–dependent protein known as calbindin-9KD. This Ca binding protein ferries the Ca across the cell cytosol to the basolateral membrane of the epithelial cell. Because the concentration of Ca inside the cell is nearly 10,000 fold lower than in the extracellular fluid, it will be necessary for the cell to pump Ca across the basolateral membrane against its electrochemical gradient in order to move the Ca into the blood. This process is achieved using a third vitamin D–dependent protein, a plasma membrane Ca-ATPase pump that uses the energy in ATP to pump Ca into the blood.[13] All 3 of these proteins are needed for the active transport of Ca across the intestinal cells and their presence within the epithelial cells depends on stimulation of the cells by $1,25(OH)_2D$. This steroid hormone has to interact with its receptor in the cell nucleus to initiate the transcription and translation of these vitamin D–dependent proteins. This process requires time. We know calbindin-9KD levels in the duodenal epithelial cells increase about 18 hours after an increase in blood $1,25(OH)_2D$,[14] and it likely takes 48 hours for full implementation of transcellular active transport of Ca processes to significantly increase blood Ca once stimulated by $1,25(OH)_2D$ in the cow.[15]

Paracellular Intestinal Ca Absorption

A second vitamin D–independent mechanism for the absorption of Ca also exists. This mechanism involves movement of Ca from the lumen of the intestine to the extracellular fluids *between* intestinal epithelial cells. This mechanism is known as paracellular Ca transport, and the mechanism is driven purely by the concentration of soluble Ca reaching the epithelial cells. When ionized Ca concentration in proximity to the tight junctions between epithelial cells significantly exceeds the ionized Ca concentration in the extracellular fluid (~ 1.25 mM), Ca flows across the tight junctions directly into the extracellular fluid and blood.[13] The following calculations can illustrate the contribution made by passive absorption of diet Ca. Let us assume a dry cow is consuming 14 kg dry matter (DM) per day of a diet that is 0.5% Ca (as low in Ca as most dry cow diets can be made), and she is drinking 35 kg of water per day.[16] We can estimate the total Ca concentration in the ingesta has been diluted to a concentration close to 30 mM. However, it is unlikely all 30 mM is in an ionized form. In a diet that is just 0.5% Ca, forages supply most of the Ca in the diet; it is likely that only 30% of this Ca is in an absorbable form.[16] Applying this factor, it is possible that the concentration of ionized Ca concentration in the ingesta could approach 10 mM. However, the presence of proteins and other chelators of free minerals within the ingesta likely reduce this estimate further. In monogastric animals, it is estimated that 30% to 60% of Ca absorbed from the diet is absorbed by the paracellular route, being closer to 30% when diet Ca is low and 60% with higher Ca levels in the diet. In cows, particularly the periparturient cow, the relative contribution of paracellular versus transcellular transport of Ca to total diet Ca absorption is unknown, though the contribution of active vitamin D–dependent transport is known to be critical when dietary Ca is low and paracellular transport becomes the more predominant pathway when dietary Ca is high (with rations containing closer to 1% diet Ca).

WHY DOES CA HOMEOSTASIS FAIL IN SOME COWS?

In most cows, the sudden exodus of Ca from the blood to support milk production is successfully met by reducing urine Ca excretion, increasing the removal of Ca from bone fluid and bone crystals, and extraction of Ca from the diet by both passive and vitamin D–dependent transport mechanisms.

At one time, it was thought milk fever occurred as a result of the failure of the parathyroid glands to recognize and respond to the hypocalcemia induced by the onset of lactation.[17] However, it was later discovered that cows developing milk fever have very high concentrations of PTH in their blood.[18] In a landmark study, Martig and Mayer[19] were able to demonstrate that the response of late-gestation cows to exogenous PTH (which should cause an increase in blood Ca concentration) was diminished compared with the response elicited by PTH administered to cows in lactation; however, they were not able to discern the cause. In severe cases of relapsing milk fever (cows relapsing and becoming recumbent again some hours after the typical intravenous Ca treatment), it was observed that the secreted PTH in these cows fails to stimulate the production of 1,25(OH)$_2$D to the same extent it does in cows with less severe milk fever (cows that require only a single intravenous Ca treatment to effect a recovery). This finding again suggested that the periparturient cow's tissues were temporarily refractory to PTH stimulation.[20] Experimental studies have identified several factors that interfere with Ca homeostasis in the cow. These factors are discussed later along with measures that can be taken to overcome their effects.

HIGH DCAD

Elegant work by Norwegian researchers Ender and colleagues[21] and Dishington[22] in the late 1960s demonstrated that reducing the dietary cation-anion difference (DCAD), defined as the difference in the number of milliequivalents of cations (primarily potassium [K$^+$] and sodium [Na$^+$]) and anions (primarily chloride [Cl$^-$] and sulfate [SO$_4^{-2}$]) in the precalving diet, improved Ca homeostasis at the onset of lactation. Block[23] was able to confirm and extend this observation. Goff and Horst[24] demonstrated that high dietary K induced a metabolic alkalosis and found the risk of developing severe periparturient hypocalcemia was greatest in those cows in a state of metabolic alkalosis. Similar results were observed when Na was added to the prepartum diet. A recent study fed late-gestation cows a high DCAD, alkalinizing diet or a low DCAD, acidifying diet and treated the cows with synthetic exogenous PTH. The cows fed the alkalinizing diet had a greatly diminished response to the PTH as compared with cows fed the acidifying diet. Their kidneys did not produce as much 1,25(OH)$_2$D, and serum Ca did not increase as quickly.[25] The researchers speculated that the tertiary structure of the PTH receptor is altered during metabolic alkalosis, reducing its affinity for PTH and resulting in a state of pseudohypoparathyroidism (see **Fig. 2B**). In many cows, despite the fact that bone and kidney cells are exposed to very high concentrations of PTH at the onset of lactation, they respond poorly to the PTH. The addition of dietary anions to counteract cations in the diet of a cow reduces the alkalinity of the blood and restores tissue responsiveness to PTH at the onset of lactation. Most studies have found physiologic functions stimulated by PTH, such as osteoclastic bone resorption and production of 1,25(OH)$_2$D, were enhanced in cows fed diets with added anions.[26–30] However, not all studies demonstrate an increase in osteoclast activity when cows are fed anionic diets.[31]

Acidifying the blood by reducing diet K and adding anions may have other effects that could help the cow restore blood Ca to normal levels. Acidification increases the amount of Ca excreted in the urine from 0.5 g/d to 5 or 6 g/d. The high hydrogen ion content of the glomerular filtrate interferes with the ability of the kidneys to reabsorb Ca from the filtrate, causing the increase in urinary Ca excretion. If the cow could reabsorb this Ca from the glomerular filtrate the day of calving, it could improve Ca balance (see **Fig. 1**). Unfortunately, it is not clear that this is the case. Schonewille and colleagues[32] fed anionic diets to cows and then treated them with a Ca chelator ethylenediaminetetraacetic acid (EDTA) to reduce ionized Ca in the blood and initiate endogenous PTH secretion. They observed that nearly all of the 5 to 6 g of urinary Ca excreted during acidosis could be returned to the blood (ie, almost none would be excreted in the urine), which could help the cow maintain Ca homeostasis during times of Ca stress. However, in a different model, Goff and colleagues[25] found that very little of the Ca excreted in acidic urine could be recovered to support blood Ca in cows treated with exogenous PTH. Studies also suggest that renal reabsorption of Ca does not increase in response to PTH in dogs or humans with metabolic acidosis.[33] However, if we assume anions are removed from the diet of the cow upon calving, the urine Ca would decrease just because the animal is not going to be acidotic on a high-DCAD lactating-cow diet. One might argue that the loss of 5 to 6 g of Ca every day in the urine during the dry period stimulated increased bone Ca removal or increased active transport of dietary Ca, and this adaptation to the acidifying prepartum diet allows 5 to 6 g of Ca to instead be used for Ca homeostasis because the alkaline urine in lactation will no longer necessitate the excretion of this much Ca in the urine.

Bone is a major source of buffer for the body.[34] During acidosis, hydrogen ions in the blood are exchanged for Ca cations in bone. It is estimated that the rapidly exchangeable bone fluid pool of a cow fed a high-DCAD diet contains 6 to 10 g of Ca. Inducing a metabolic acidosis in a cow increases the amount of Ca available for osteocytic osteolysis in the bone fluid pool by 5 to 6 g.[35] Braithwaite[36] studied the effect of dietary Ca chloride on bone exchangeable Ca pools in older sheep. Using his data and extrapolating it to a 600-kg cow, inducing a metabolic acidosis by dietary anion supplementation would increase bone-exchangeable Ca about 3.5 g the first week of feeding Ca chloride and up to 14 g after 10 weeks of feeding the Ca chloride. Braithewaite's data have a very high standard error, which caused him to question his results; but taken together with many other studies reported since his work, the data suggest bone fluid pool Ca content is increased by low-DCAD diets. This readily exchangeable bone Ca is likely to contribute greatly to Ca homeostasis on stimulation of the osteocytes by PTH (see **Fig. 1**). This response is fast and likely begins within minutes after PTH secretion increases, *if the tissues are not resistant to the effects of PTH*. Evidence for the critical role osteocytic osteolysis plays in Ca homeostasis response to acute hypocalcemia can be observed in studies that use the Ca chelator Na-EDTA administered intravenously to induce hypocalcemia. For instance, Wang and Beede[37] infused Na-EDTA and found that nonpregnant, nonlactating cows fed anionic diets could withstand a larger Ca stress imposed over a 3-hour period better than cows fed a high-DCAD diet. The difference was a little more than 1.1 g of Ca mobilized during the 3 hours of infusion of EDTA. The short time frame of this study and the use of nonpregnant, nonlactating cows suggest the only source capable of replacing the EDTA-bound Ca this quickly was osteocytic osteolysis of the bone fluid exchangeable pool. Osteoclastic bone resorption and vitamin D–dependent intestinal Ca absorption take much more time to activate, and passive vitamin D–independent Ca absorption should not respond to Ca stressors. Even under acidic conditions, less than 0.8 g of Ca would be excreted in the urine over the course of 3 hours; Even if all of this Ca was reabsorbed by the kidney, which is unlikely, it would not account for the improved response of the anion cows to EDTA infusion over this short time frame.

Application of DCAD Theory to Reduce Periparturient Hypocalcemia

In theory, all the cations and anions in a diet are capable of exerting an influence on the electrical charge of the blood. The major cations present in feeds and the charge they carry are Na (+1), K (+1), Ca (+2), and magnesium (Mg) (+2). The major anions and their charges found in feeds are Cl (−1), SO_4 (−2), and PO_4 (assumed to be −3). Cations or anions present in the diet will only alter the electrical charge of the blood if they are absorbed into the blood. Trace elements present in diets are absorbed in such small amounts that they are of negligible consequence to the acid-base status. Organic acids such as the volatile fatty acids are generally absorbed in the undissociated, neutral form so they carry no net charge into the blood. They are also rapidly metabolized within the liver, so when they do dissociate they have only a small effect on blood pH under most circumstances. An exception is during rumen lactic acidosis, whereby the lactate anion builds up to unusually high levels in the blood.

Desired Mineral Profile of Prepartum Diet

The difference between the number of cation and anion particles absorbed from the diet determines the pH of the blood. The cation-anion difference of a diet is commonly described in terms of milliequivalent per kilogram (some researchers prefer to use mEq/100-g diet) of just Na, K, Cl, and SO_4 (traditionally calculated on the basis of S% reported when diet is analyzed by wet chemistry) as follows:

$$DCAD = (mEq\ Na^+ + mEq\ K^+) - (mEq\ Cl^- + mEq\ SO_4^{2-}).$$

This equation is useful, although it must be kept in mind that Ca, Mg, and PO_4 absorbed from the diet will also influence blood pH. Evaluation of the relative acidifying activity of dietary Cl versus SO_4 demonstrates that SO_4 is only about 60% as acidifying as Cl.[38–40] The DCAD of a diet and its acidifying activity is more accurately described by the following equation: $(Na^+ + K^+) - (Cl^- + 0.6\ S^{2-})$. A more complex DCAD equation would include Ca, Mg, and P. It should probably also include ammonium, as this cation seems to also contribute to the cation content of the blood.[41] Unfortunately, experimental data are lacking that would allow assignment of a coefficient of absorption to each of these dietary ions when fed to the dry cow. Although DCAD equations provide a theoretical basis for dietary manipulation of the acid-base status, they are not necessary for formulation of mineral content of prepartum dairy cow rations because (with the exception of K and Cl) the rate of inclusion of the other macrominerals can be set at fixed rates.

Na

The National Research Council's (NRC)[16] requirement for Na in the diet of a late-gestation cow is about 0.12%. Feedstuffs typically used in rations for late-gestation cows generally do not supply this amount of Na. (Exceptions occur, especially when forages are grown where irrigation has led to increased salinity of the soil.) A small amount of salt is added to the diet to prevent pica, which often is manifest as a desire to drink urine from the floor. Exceeding the requirement for Na using NaCl is to be avoided in late gestation because it will increase the risk of udder edema not because it greatly affects the acid-base status.

Ca

At least 2 studies have clearly demonstrated that inclusion of Ca in the diet at the NRC-required levels or several fold more than the NRC-required levels does not influence the degree of hypocalcemia experienced by the cow at calving.[24,42] Beede and colleagues[42] fed 0.47%-, 0.98%-, 1.52%-, and 1.95%-Ca diets to cows in late gestation being fed a high-Cl diet to prevent milk fever. Cows fed 1.5%-Ca diets had slightly reduced feed intake when compared with control cows, whereas those fed the 1.95%-Ca diet had significantly lower feed intake. Dietary Ca did not influence the degree of hypocalcemia experienced at calving or milk production in the subsequent lactation. It seems from this study that a close-up dietary Ca concentration of 1% is optimal. This Ca level is similar to the level the cow will receive in the lactating diet; Feeding a higher diet Ca may contribute even more Ca to the blood via the paracellular route, however, higher dietary Ca could also negatively impact feed intake.

Mg

To ensure adequate concentrations of Mg in the blood of the periparturient cow, the dietary Mg concentration should be 0.35% to 0.4% to take advantage of passive absorption of Mg across the rumen wall. This point is particularly important in the prepartum and early lactation diets. Further, hypomagnesemia is the primary cause of midlactation milk fever in cows. The pathophysiology behind this is discussed in detail in the section on Mg.

P

Dietary P concentration should meet but not exceed the NRC's requirement for P in the late-gestation cow. This concentration is generally about 0.35% P for most cows, though recent studies suggest this may still overestimate the true requirement of the cow for dietary P.[43] Because phosphate is an anion, one might consider using phosphate to acidify the blood. Unfortunately, this is likely to cause milk fever. When blood P concentration is increased to the upper end of the normal limit, around 6 mg/100 mL (1.9 mM), the phosphate has a direct inhibitory effect on the renal enzyme that converts 25-OH vitamin D to $1,25(OH)_2D$. Therefore, even if PTH secretion occurs and the tissues recognize the PTH, the cow will be unable to produce the $1,25(OH)_2D$ necessary for transcellular intestinal Ca transport and will suffer impaired Ca homeostasis.[44,45] A diet supplying more than 80 g of P per day greatly increases the risk of milk fever. Keeping dietary P less than 50 g/d seems to be safe, though lower levels (35 g/d) improve Ca homeostasis.[43] Keeping dietary P low in the prepartum diet does not contribute to the hypophosphatemic downer cow condition, which is sometimes observed as a sequela of milk fever.[46]

S

Dietary S must be kept greater than 0.22% (to ensure adequate substrate for rumen microbial amino acid synthesis) but less than 0.4% (to avoid possible neurologic problems associated with S toxicity).[47] Ca sulfate and Mg sulfate are good sources of S that may also supply any needed Mg and Ca. The author prefers close up diets that contain 0.35-0.4% S. Sulfuric acid may also be used to increase dietary S to 0.4% if proper handling precautions are observed, which includes a respirator as the fumes are very hazardous.

K and Cl

Now, with the exception of K and Cl, the variables in the proposed DCAD equations have become fixed. The key to milk fever prevention (Holstein cows) is to keep K as close to the NRC's requirement of the dry cow as possible (about 1.0% diet K). The key to the reduction of subclinical hypocalcemia, not just milk fever prevention, is to add Cl⁻ anions to the ration to counteract the effects of low diet K on blood alkalinity. For formulation purposes, the concentration of Cl required in the diet to acidify the cow should first be set at 0.5% less than the concentration of K in the diet. In other words, if dietary K can be reduced to 1.3%, the Cl concentration of the diet should be increased to 0.8%. This level of chloride will adequately acidify about 20% of herds in this author's experience. Ultimately, in many herds, the amount of chloride added will have to be brought to within 0.25 to 0.3% of the dietary K for proper acidification. A conservative approach should be taken when formulating the diet of close-up cows, as going immediately to the higher chloride diet will cause overacidification of 20% of herds. Overacidification can reduce feed intake, creating many other metabolic disease challenges. Move to the higher dose of chloride only if urine acidification (described as a monitoring tool later) is not achieved at the lower chloride level. There is also a limit on how much anion can be added to a diet without affecting feed intake. In this author's experience, when diet K exceeds 1.4%, it is difficult to add enough chloride to the diet using the traditional chloride salts (Ca, ammonium, and Mg chloride) to acidify the cow and maintain adequate dry matter intake. With some of the more palatable commercial anion supplements, it is possible to acidify the diets and maintain feed intake when dietary K is as high as 1.8%. If dietary K can only be reduced to 2.0%, the Cl would need to be roughly 1.5% to acidify the cow. Increasing Cl to this level in the diet is likely to cause a decrease in dry matter intake. Chloride and sulfate sources differ in their palatability; because achieving low dietary K can be difficult, it is prudent to use a palatable source of Cl or sulfate when formulating the diet. Ammonium chloride (or ammonium sulfate) can be particularly unpalatable when included in rations with a high pH. At the higher pH of high forage (low corn silage) rations whereby the pH of the diet exceeds 5.5, the ammonium cation is converted to ammonia, which is highly irritating when smelled by the cow. Prilling the Cl (and SO_4) salts can reduce the unpleasant taste of the salts and allow improved anion supplementation success. In this author's experience, hydrochloric acid has proved to be the most palatable source of anions as well as the strongest acidifying agent. However, hydrochloric acid can be extremely dangerous to handle when it is procured as a liquid concentrate. Several companies now manufacture anion supplements composed of hydrochloric acid adsorbed onto feed particles, which are safe to handle and palatable.

Monitoring Urine pH

These are simply guidelines for anion supplementation used by this author and are based on the inclusion of Ca, Na, S, Mg, and P at the levels outlined earlier. Urine pH of the cow provides a cheap and fairly accurate assessment of blood pH and can be a good gauge of the appropriate level of anion supplementation.[48] Urine pH on high-cation diets is generally more than 8.2. Limiting dietary cations will reduce urine pH only a small amount (down to 7.5–7.8). For optimal control of subclinical hypocalcemia, the average pH of the urine of Holstein cows should be between 6.2 and 6.8 during the last week of gestation, which essentially requires the addition of anions to the ration. In Jersey cows, the average urine pH of the close-up cows has to be reduced to between 5.8 and 6.3 for effective control of hypocalcemia. If the average urine pH is between 5.0 and 5.5, excessive anions have been added and there is the danger they have induced an uncompensated metabolic acidosis; the cows will suffer a decline in dry matter intake, even if a palatable anion supplement is used. Urine pH should be checked 72 or more hours after a ration change. Urine samples should be free of feces and made on midstream collections to avoid alkalinity contributed by vaginal secretions. The best estimate of acid-base status seems to be from samples obtained 6 to 9 hours after fresh feed is offered. The timing of urine collection is less critical than adopting the habit of regularly checking urine pH of cows in the last week of gestation. Anion-supplemented diets are generally fed for the last 3 to 4 weeks before calving. If anions are fed the entire dry period, be aware that after 3 weeks on anion diets, urine pH will begin to move toward neutral as the bone buffers the acidity brought in with the anions. The author's experience is that the diet remains effective, but the use of urine pH in the final week of gestation will become inaccurate. Over time, the urine pH will have increased by 0.5 to 0.75 pH units. The recommendation of this author is to use urine pH determinations made on cows that have been on the diet 2 to 3 weeks as the gauge of whether sufficient anions have been added to the diet.

Agronomic Considerations for Producing Low DCAD Forages

Reducing K in the ration of the late-gestation cow can present a problem.[49] All plants need a certain amount of K for maximal growth. Corn is a warm-season grass and grows maximally when plant tissue is 1.1% to 1.5% K, making corn silage a low K choice for dry cows. However, the corn grain accompanying the silage may supply more energy than desired in a dry cow diet. Other warm-season (prairie) grasses, such as switchgrass, big bluestem, and Indiangrass, are low in K but are also low in energy. Legumes and cool-season grasses are poor choices for dry cow diets as they accumulate K within their tissues to concentrations that are well above that required for optimal growth (2.0%–2.2%). Alfalfa grown on farms fertilized with manure is generally greater than 3% K. If cool-season grasses and legumes contain less than 2% K, it is likely the yield suffered. When liquid manure is applied to the land, it brings large amounts of K to the soil and relatively small amounts of Cl. Forages become very high in DCAD. If KCl (potash) is used to meet the K needs of the plants, the DCAD may not be severely high as the K taken up within the plant is often accompanied by Cl. It is possible to find hays that are low in K and high (1.0%–1.2%) in Cl.[50,51] Producers should use the lowest DCAD forage possible not simply the lowest K forage. Keep in mind that a low DCAD forage is not useful if it is unpalatable; highly mature forages, corn stover, and forages rained on during the drying process are low in K but are less palatable. Producers should routinely analyze for both K and Cl in forages. Traditional wet chemistry analyses are preferred as near-infrared spectroscopy is a notoriously poor way to determine mineral content.

HYPOMAGNESEMIA

Insufficient dietary Mg supply leads to hypomagnesemia. Hypomagnesemia is a major risk factor for milk fever.[52,53] van Mosel and colleagues[52] also demonstrated that the ability to absorb dietary Mg declined with age, increasing the risk of developing hypomagnesemia. Hypomagnesemia affects Ca metabolism in 2 major ways.

1. By reducing tissue sensitivity to PTH: As already discussed in the DCAD section, the integrity of the interaction between PTH and its receptor is vital to Ca homeostasis. Hypomagnesemia is also capable of interfering with the ability of PTH to act on its target tissues. Prolonged hypomagnesemia (days) causes a decline in intracellular as well as extracellular Mg concentration.[54] The adenylyl cyclase enzyme has a binding site for Mg, and the evidence from in vitro studies suggests the lack of an Mg ion will not permit adenylyl cyclase to convert Mg ATP to cyclic AMP (see **Fig. 2**C). It is clear that ATP and GTP must be complexed with an Mg ion in order to stabilize their shape so they can fit into the catalytic sites of most enzymes. It is less clear whether intracellular Mg levels could decline to levels that limit the availability of these compounds and block ATP- or GTP-dependent functions in the cells. In humans, it is well recognized that chronic hypomagnesemia can cause hypocalcemia and that Mg therapy alone restores the serum Ca concentration to normal; Ca and/or vitamin D therapy are ineffective.[55] Blood Mg concentrations less than 1.6 mg/dL in the periparturient cow will increase the susceptibility of cows to hypocalcemia and milk fever.[56]

2. By reducing PTH secretion in response to hypocalcemia: PTH secretion is normally increased greatly in response to even slight decreases in blood Ca concentration. However, the Ca-sensing receptor on the parathyroid gland cells is a G-protein coupled receptor. Insufficient absorption of dietary Mg results in a decline in extracellular and intracellular Mg concentration. It is thought that the depletion of intracellular Mg interferes with the ability of the G-α protein to interact with adenylyl cyclase and for the adenylyl cyclase to effectively convert Mg-ATP to cyclic AMP, and so PTH secretion is not initiated.[57,58] In cattle, blood Mg must be less than 1.4 mg/dL for a period of time for this blockade of PTH secretion to occur. This requirement seems to be a factor in the development of some hypomagnesemic tetany syndromes of grazing beef and dairy cattle. A report on lactating beef cows grazing tetany-prone pastures demonstrated that plasma Mg concentrations declined slowly over several weeks, with plasma Mg concentrations between 0.8 and 1.4 mg/dL in most of the cows who remained asymptomatic. However, in those animals exhibiting clinical disease (tetany), blood Ca had also decreased and was less than 5 mg/dL. In other words, tetany only occurred when both plasma Mg and Ca concentrations declined. Blood Ca concentration had remained within normal limits the day before the animals developed tetany but had decreased precipitously that day. Plasma PTH concentrations did not increase as a result of the decline in blood Ca concentration, and the researchers concluded that hypomagnesemia had blocked PTH secretion preventing the cows from maintaining normal Ca homeostasis.[59]

FEEDING A LOW-CA DIET BEFORE CALVING TO PREVENT HYPOCALCEMIA

If cows are fed a diet that supplies less Ca than they require before calving, and placed on a high-Ca diet immediately after calving, hypocalcemia and milk fever can be prevented. If the prepartum diet supplies less absorbable Ca than the tissues require, the cow goes into negative Ca balance. This negative Ca balance causes a minor decline in blood Ca concentration stimulating PTH secretion. Prolonged exposure to elevated PTH can stimulate osteoclastic bone resorption and renal production of 1,25(OH)$_2$D within 1 to 2 weeks of the diet change *even in the face of metabolic alkalosis induced by a high-DCAD diet*. This stimulation increases daily bone Ca efflux and prepares the intestine to absorb Ca efficiently via transcellular transport of Ca once Ca is supplied in the lactating ration.[45,60,61] The studies that demonstrated this strategy would work fed less than 20 g of Ca per cow per day. Few farms in the United States today can formulate diets that supply less than 50 g of Ca per cow per day, and this is not sufficiently low enough to stimulate PTH secretion prepartum.

The absorbed Ca requirement of the late-gestation cow is from 14 g/d in Jerseys to about 22 g in large Holsteins.[16] A truly low-Ca diet capable of stimulating PTH secretion supplies considerably less absorbable Ca than required by the cow.[60,61] A 600-kg cow consuming 13 kg of DM must be fed a diet that is less than 0.15% absorbable Ca if it is to provide less than 20 g of available Ca per day. Low-Ca diets have proven more practical under grazing situations. In these cases, the total dry matter intake of pasture was 6 to 7 kg of DM per day and the grasses being grazed were less than 0.4% Ca, which would provide less than 28 g of total Ca and somewhere around 9 to 10 g of absorbable Ca per day (Sanchez JM, personal communication, 2003, University of Costa Rica, San Jose, Costa Rica). It is important to note that after calving, the animal must be switched to a high-Ca diet for this strategy to succeed.

Recently, a method has been developed to reduce the availability of dietary Ca for absorption. It involves incorporation of zeolite (a silicate particle) into the ration, which binds

Ca and causes it to be passed out in the feces. The original research describing this method used a form of zeolite that was unwieldy because very large amounts of zeolite had to be ingested each day ($\sim$ 1 kg). In addition, the effects of zeolite on P and trace mineral absorption were not clear.[62] At present, an improved form of zeolite is commercially available in Europe. By chemically modifying the zeolite, the affinity and the specificity of the zeolite for Ca have been improved so that an effective dose of the commercial preparation is approaching 0.5 kg/d. It is still essential to use a low-Ca diet prepartum and to add Mg to the diet. It is also critical to switch to a high-Ca lactation diet at calving.

VITAMIN D SUPPLEMENTATION

A reasonable practice is to supplement the dry cow with 20,000 to 35,000 IU of vitamin D per day. This amount increases serum 25-OH vitamin D concentrations to levels from 30 to 50 ng/mL providing adequate substrate for the synthesis of 1,25(OH)$_2$D. Earlier literature often recommended feeding or injecting massive doses (up to 10 million units of vitamin D) 10 to 14 days before calving to prevent milk fever.[63,64] The vitamin D is converted to 25-OH vitamin D. Blood levels of 25-OH vitamin D become very high and at these levels it begins to bind to and activate the VDR, just as 1,25(OH)$_2$D does. This action will pharmacologically increase intestinal Ca absorption and can help prevent milk fever. Unfortunately, the dose of vitamin D that effectively prevents milk fever is very close to the level that causes irreversible metastatic calcification of soft tissues. Lower doses (500,000 to 1 million units of vitamin D) may actually induce milk fever because the high levels of 25-OH vitamin D resulting from treatment suppress PTH secretion and directly suppress renal synthesis of endogenous 1,25(OH)$_2$D.[64] The animals become hypocalcemic when the exogenous source of vitamin D that had maintained elevated intestinal Ca absorption rates is cleared from the body. When massive doses of vitamin D are administered, the ability to synthesize 1,25(OH)$_2$D in the cow's kidney is severely suppressed. In some cases, this prevents hypocalcemia at calving, but causes a severe delayed hypocalcemia to occur 7 to 12 days after calving.[64]

Treatment with 1,25(OH)$_2$D and its analogues can be more effective and much safer than using vitamin D, but problems associated with the timing of administration remain.[65,66] The problem of suppression of renal 1,25(OH)$_2$D production can be minimized by slow withdrawal of the exogenous hormone over a period of days after calving.[67] These more potent vitamin D compounds are not available for use in the United States.

ORAL CA TREATMENTS AT CALVING

Ca administered to the fresh cow may arguably be called a treatment rather than a preventative measure for hypocalcemia. Contrasts between the effects observed with intravenous, subcutaneous, and oral Ca treatments have been described elsewhere.[68,69] Briefly, the concept behind oral supplementation is that the cow's ability to use active transport of Ca across intestinal cells is inadequate to help her maintain normal blood Ca concentrations. By dosing the animal with large amounts of very soluble Ca, it is possible to force Ca across the intestinal tract by means of passive diffusion between intestinal epithelial cells. The best results are obtained with doses of Ca between 50 and 90 g of Ca per dose. Ca chloride has been used but can be very caustic. Ca propionate is less injurious to tissues and has the added benefit of supplying propionate, a gluconeogenic precursor. Ca carbonate is not soluble enough to induce a rapid increase in blood Ca. For best control of hypocalcemia, a dose is given at calving and again 24 hours later. Toxic doses of Ca can be delivered orally; a single dose of 250 g of Ca in a soluble form will kill some cows.[70] The benefit of adding oral Ca drenches/gels in addition to a properly formulated low-DCAD program is becoming easier to justify as recent studies link even moderate hypocalcemia with decreased health and performance of the cow.[4,5,71] For 2 to 3 hours after these treatments are administered, the concentration of ionized Ca in the fluids within the rumen and small intestine is high enough (4-6 mM Ca) to drive Ca into the blood by the paracellular route until the ionized Ca concentration at the absorptive surfaces decreases below 4-6 mM Ca. It has been estimated that about 4 g of Ca entered the blood of cows given 50 g of Ca as Ca chloride in a drench in the first hours following treatment.[72]

AGE

Older cows have greater difficulty maintaining Ca homeostasis than young cows, especially as they progress to the third or greater lactation. With advancing age, there is a reduction in the number of receptors for 1,25(OH)$_2$D in the intestine of cows.[73] In addition, once the cow reaches a mature skeletal size (toward the end of the first lactation), the number of active sites of bone remodeling is reduced. This reduction means there are fewer active osteoclasts and osteoblasts present on bone surfaces. When PTH is secreted in response to hypocalcemia in the older cow, there will be fewer osteoblasts to respond to it; it will also require a greater length of time to achieve osteoclastic bone resorption as new osteoclasts must be recruited from osteoclast progenitors and then activated to resorb bone. In the first calf heifer, the osteoclasts are present and need only be activated by PTH. There is also evidence that the number of PTH receptors in the kidney declines with age.[74] Perhaps this also occurs in aged osteoblasts and osteocytes.

BREED

The Jersey and, to a lesser extent, the *Swedish Red* and *White* and *Norwegian Red* breeds are well known to have a higher incidence of milk fever compared with Holstein cows. Jersey cow colostrum and true milk have higher concentrations of Ca than Holstein colostrum and milk. However, when the higher milk and colostrum production of Holsteins is taken into account the Ca drain imposed per kg of body weight is only slightly greater in Jersey cows. A 15% reduction in the number of receptors for 1,25(OH)$_2$D in intestinal tissues of Jerseys versus Holsteins has been observed, but there was a large standard error to these measurements.[75] It is reported that Holsteins and Brown Swiss have similar amounts of 1,25(OH)$_2$D receptors in their intestinal tract.[76]

Summary of Hypocalcemia Avoidance Measures

At the onset of lactation, all cows go into negative Ca balance; they must draw on bone reserves of Ca and maximize the use of the Ca in their diet (mediated by 1,25[OH]2D) to avoid hypocalcemia. Reducing urinary Ca losses can also be helpful. The key to successful Ca homeostasis is bone and kidney tissue that is capable of responding to PTH. Metabolic alkalosis caused by high-DCAD diets prevents PTH from interacting strongly with its receptor, blocking osteocytic osteolysis (rapid Ca release) and osteoclastic (slower but greater magnitude) bone resorption. High-DCAD diets also prevent renal production of 1,25(OH)$_2$D preventing the use of the active transcellular absorption of Ca across the intestine. Hypomagnesemia causes intracellular ionized Mg to decline; adenylyl cyclase, which requires Mg^{++} as a cofactor, fails to produce cyclic AMP in response to PTH stimulation, again causing hypocalcemia. Prolonged PTH stimulation can overcome the effects of high-DCAD diets on the PTH receptor affinity for PTH. However, it cannot overcome the effects of hypomagnesemia. Low-Ca diets (<25 g of Ca per day) could stimulate PTH secretion for a prolonged period before calving, but these diets are difficult to formulate. High-Ca diets after calving or Ca drenches/gels administered at calving take advantage of passive paracellular Ca absorption to restore blood Ca to normal levels.

MG
Body Content and Distribution of Mg

Mg is a major intracellular cation that is a necessary cofactor for enzymatic reactions vital to every major metabolic pathway. Extracellular Mg is vital to normal nerve conduction, muscle function, and bone mineral formation. Cow plasma Mg concentration is normally between 1.9 and 2.4 mg/dL (0.80 and 1.0 mmol/L). Approximately 20% of this is protein bound; 65% is ionized; and the rest is complexed with various anions, such as phosphate and citrate. Acid base disturbances (metabolic acidosis or alkalosis) have little effect on the distribution of serum Mg. The concentration of Mg in cerebrospinal fluid (CSF) is around 2.4 mg/dL, of which 55% is free and 45% is complexed with other compounds. In a 600-kg cow, there is about 0.85 g of Mg in the blood, 3 g of Mg in all extracellular fluids, 79 g of Mg inside cells, and 205 g of Mg within bone mineral.[77] Bone is not a significant source of Mg that can be used in times of Mg deficit, as bone resorption occurs in response to Ca homeostasis not Mg status. The maintenance of normal plasma Mg concentration is nearly totally dependent on dietary Mg absorption. A reduction in serum Mg concentration increases excitability of nervous tissue. Because extracellular and intracellular Mg are in equilibrium, prolonged (more than 1 or 2 days), hypomagnesemia reduces intracellular Mg and interferes with adenylyl cyclase activity; this can interfere with many metabolic responses as described earlier.[54] Hypomagnesemic tetany is caused by uncontrolled activation of peripheral nerves and is likely to be observed when serum Mg concentrations decrease less than 1.2 mg/dL. Seizures and convulsions occur when the cerebrospinal fluid Mg concentration decreases less than 1 mg/dL.[68]

Mg is well absorbed from the small intestine of young calves and lambs. As the rumen and reticulum develop, these sites become the main, and perhaps the only, sites for net Mg absorption.[78–81] In adult ruminants, the small intestine is a site of net secretion of Mg.[82] Mg absorption from the rumen depends on the concentration of Mg in solution in the rumen fluid and the integrity of the Mg transport mechanism, which is a Na-linked active transport process.[83]

Factors Affecting the Soluble Mg Content in the Rumen

The soluble concentration of Mg in rumen fluid depends on

- Dietary Mg content: Low Mg forages and inadequate supplementation keep soluble Mg concentrations in rumen fluid low.
- The pH of the rumen fluid: Mg solubility declines sharply as rumen pH increases above 6.5. Grazing animals have higher rumen pH because of the high K content of pasture and the stimulation of salivary buffer secretion associated with grazing. In addition, heavily fertilized, lush pastures are often high in nonprotein nitrogen and relatively low in readily fermentable carbohydrates. The ability of the rumen microbes to incorporate the nonprotein nitrogen into microbial protein is exceeded; ammonia and ammonium ions build up in the rumen, increasing pH. When high grain rations are fed, rumen fluid pH is often less than pH 6.5, increasing Mg solubility and availability.
- Mg binders within forage: Forages often contain 100 to 200 mmol/kg of unsaturated palmitic, linoleic, and linolenic acids, which can form insoluble Mg salts in

the rumen. Plants also can contain transaconitic acid. A metabolite of transaconitic acid, tricarballylate can complex Mg and is resistant to rumen degradation and may play a role in hypomagnesemic tetany in grazing cows.[84]

Factors Affecting Active Transport of Mg Across the Rumen

Forages and pastures are generally fairly low in Na. Adding Na to the ration can improve Mg transport across the rumen when dietary Na is less than the requirements; though in high amounts, it increases urinary excretion of Mg so that the benefit to the animal may be negated. High dietary K can reduce the absorption of Mg.[85] Newton and colleagues[86] fed lambs either a low-K diet (0.6% K) or high-K diet (4.9% K) and found about a 50% reduction in apparent Mg absorption. High K concentration in the rumen fluid depolarizes the apical membrane of the rumen epithelium reducing the electromotive potential needed to drive Mg across the rumen wall. The negative effects of a high-K diet cannot be overcome by adding extra Na to the diet.[83] Feeding ionophores (monensin, lasalocid) can improve activity of the Na-linked Mg transport system in the rumen, increasing Mg absorption efficiency about 10%.[82] However, ionophores are not always approved for use in many of the animals they could benefit. Lush high-moisture pastures can also increase the rate of passage of Mg from the rumen reducing the amount absorbed.

Using Other Transport Mechanisms to Absorb Dietary Mg

The active transport mechanism for Mg absorption across the rumen wall is critical to the survival of the animal when the dietary Mg concentration is less than 0.25%. Unfortunately, there are several known factors, such as dietary K, and several unknown factors that prevent efficient Mg absorption by this pathway. A second pathway for absorption of Mg exists that operates only at high rumen fluid Mg concentrations. At high rumen Mg concentration, the Mg will flow paracellularly down its concentration gradient into the extracellular fluids of the cow.[83] This passive transport mechanism is not subject to poisoning by K and is only dependent on the solubility of the Mg in the rumen.

The concentration of ionized Mg in rumen fluid needed to use the concentration gradient driven absorption of Mg is greater than 4 mmol/L.[81,85,86] The minimum level of Mg required in the diet to prevent a negative Mg balance in the face of high K levels in ruminants is approximately 0.35%.[85] Mg content of the close-up dry cow ration and the early lactation ration should be between 0.35% and 0.4% as insurance against the possibility that the active transport processes for Mg absorption are impaired.

Assessing Mg Status at Parturition

When the diet is adequate in absorbable Mg, the kidneys excrete the excess. PTH causes increased renal tubular reabsorption of Mg, so the kidneys excrete less Mg; this causes blood Mg to be elevated in the typical milk fever cow.[9,83] However, if dietary Mg is insufficient or rumen absorption of Mg is impaired, there is not enough Mg absorbed into the blood to even reach the normal renal threshold for Mg. Sampling the blood of several cows within 12 hours after calving is a simple, effective index of Mg status of the periparturient cow. If serum Mg concentration is not at least 2.0 mg/dL in 9 of 10 cows sampled, it suggests inadequate dietary Mg absorption from either a lack of diet Mg or interferences with absorption. This same test can be used in the first weeks of lactation to see if the lactating cow's diet is providing adequate Mg to the animal. Hypomagnesemia may be limiting the productivity of lactating cows by causing inefficiencies in energy metabolism as it may be limiting the availability of Mg-ATP. As mentioned earlier, hypomagnesemia can be a cause of hypocalcemia.

In this author's experience, more than 75% of midlactation milk fever cases are the result of inadequate dietary Mg in the lactating cow's diet. It is also the author's experience that the availability of Mg from the Mg oxide (MgO) used in lactating rations is often insufficient. The treatment of hypomagnesemic cows is described extensively in other reviews.[68]

Assessing Availability of Mg from Mineral Sources

Mg is included in dairy rations for 2 reasons: to maintain adequate levels of Mg in the blood and as a rumen fluid alkalinizer. Mg sulfate.7 H_2O and Mg chloride.2 H_2O are very soluble, very available sources of Mg, though they are also relatively low in Mg being just 9% and 18% Mg respectively, as the common Mg salts are highly hydrated. Mg sulfate and Mg chloride are not very palatable either. They are also not going to provide any rumen buffering action in lactating diets. Mg oxide (MgO) takes up little room in the ration, costs less, and is more palatable than some other sources of Mg. It is alkalinizing, not acidifying, so it is more appropriately used in lactation diets. The feed industry uses MgO, which is about 54% to 56% Mg. (When MgO contains more than 56% Mg it often indicates the ore was overly heated in the calcining process and the Mg will be poorly available.) Unfortunately, there is tremendous variability in MgO bioavailability. For ruminants, MgO should be ground to a fine dust. A quick test can estimate the relative availability of MgO sources. Place 3 g of an MgO source in a container and slowly add 40 mL of 5% acetic acid (white vinegar). Cap the container and shake well for 15 seconds, and let it sit. Check the pH after 30 minutes. Vinegar alone has a pH of 2.6 to 2.8. The best MgO sources will bring the pH up to 8.2 and the worst to just 3.8. pH is a log scale, so this represents greater than a 3000-fold difference in the number of hydrogen ions buffered. Remember in lactating rations, MgO is relied on to combat rumen acidosis; we are not getting that action from these insoluble MgO sources. In an experiment with 4 cows with rumen fistulas, the solubility of MgO in vitro (tested in various ways) was found to parallel their solubility in the rumen and their urinary excretion.[87,88]

REFERENCES

1. USDA National Animal Health Monitoring Survey: Dairy 2007. Part I: reference of dairy cattle health and management practices in the United States, USDA-NAHMS Technical Bulletin 2007. p. 84.
2. Reinhardt TA, Lippolis JD, McCluskey BJ, et al. Prevalence of subclinical hypocalcemia in dairy herds. Vet J 2011;188(1):122–4.
3. Kimura K, Reinhardt TA, Goff JP. Parturition and hypocalcemia blunts calcium signals in immune cells of dairy cattle. J Dairy Sci 2006;89(7):2588–95.
4. Martinez N, Risco CA, Lima FS, et al. Evaluation of peripartal calcium status, energetic profile, and neutrophil function in dairy cows at low or high risk of developing uterine disease. J Dairy Sci 2012;95(12):7158–72.
5. Chamberlin WG, Middleton JR, Spain JN, et al. Subclinical hypocalcemia, plasma biochemical parameters, lipid metabolism, postpartum disease, and fertility in postparturient dairy cows. J Dairy Sci 2013;96(11):7001–13.
6. Brown EM. Clinical lessons from the calcium-sensing receptor. Nat Clin Pract Endocrinol Metab 2007;3(2):122–33.
7. Potts JT, Gardella TJ. Progress, paradox, and potential: parathyroid hormone research over five decades. Ann N Y Acad Sci 2007;1117:196–208.
8. Hoorn EJ, Zietse R. Disorders of calcium and magnesium balance: a physiology-based approach. Pediatr Nephrol 2013;28(8):1195–206.

9. Goff JP, Littledike ET, Horst RL. Effect of synthetic bovine parathyroid hormone in dairy cows: prevention of hypocalcemic parturient paresis. J Dairy Sci 1986; 69(9):2278–89.

10. Teti A, Zallone A. Do osteocytes contribute to bone mineral homeostasis? Osteocytic osteolysis revisited. Bone 2009;44(1):11–6.

11. Ward G, Harbers LH, Blaha JJ. Calcium-containing crystals in alfalfa: their fate in cattle. J Dairy Sci 1979;62(5):715–22.

12. Martz FA, Belo AT, Weiss MF, et al. True absorption of calcium and phosphorus from alfalfa and corn silage when fed to lactating cows. J Dairy Sci 1990;73(5): 1288–95.

13. Christakos S. Recent advances in our understanding of 1,25-dihydroxyvitamin D(3) regulation of intestinal calcium absorption. Arch Biochem Biophys 2012; 523(1):73–6.

14. Wasserman RH, Fullmer CS. Vitamin D and intestinal calcium transport: facts, speculations and hypotheses. J Nutr 1995;125(Suppl 7):1971S–9S.

15. Goff JP, Horst RL, Littledike ET, et al. Bone resorption, renal function and mineral status in cows treated with 1,25-dihydroxycholecalciferol and its 24-fluoro analogues. J Nutr 1986;116(8):1500–10.

16. National Research Council. Nutrient requirements of dairy cattle. Washington, DC: National Academy Press; 2000.

17. Capen CC, Young DM. The ultrastructure of the parathyroid glands and thyroid parafollicular cells of cows with parturient paresis and hypocalcemia. Lab Invest 1967;17(6):717–37.

18. Mayer GP, Ramberg CF Jr, Kronfeld DS, et al. Plasma parathyroid hormone concentration in hypocalcemic parturient cows. Am J Vet Res 1969;30(9):1587–97.

19. Martig J, Mayer GP. Diminished hypercalcemic response to parathyroid extract in prepartum cows. J Dairy Sci 1973;56(8):1042–6.

20. Goff JP, Reinhardt TA, Horst RL. Recurring hypocalcemia of bovine parturient paresis is associated with failure to produce 1,25-dihydroxyvitamin D. Endocrinology 1989;125(1):49–53.

21. Ender F, Dishington IW, Helgebostad A. Calcium balance studies in dairy cows under experimental induction and prevention of hypocalcaemic paresis puerperalis. The solution of the aetiology and the prevention of milk fever by dietary means. Z Tierphysiol 1971;28:233–56.

22. Dishington IW. Prevention of milk fever (hypocalcemic paresis puerperalis) by dietary salt supplements. Acta Vet Scand 1975;16(4):503–12.

23. Block E. Manipulating dietary anions and cations for prepartum dairy cows to reduce incidence of milk fever. J Dairy Sci 1984;67:2939–48.

24. Goff JP, Horst RL. Effects of the addition of potassium or sodium, but not calcium, to prepartum ratios on milk fever in dairy cows. J Dairy Sci 1997;80(1):176–86.

25. Goff JP, Liesegang A, Horst RL. Diet induced pseudohypoparathyroidism: a milk fever risk factor. J Dairy Sci 2014;97(3):1520–8.

26. Leclerc H, Block E. Effects of reducing dietary cation-anion balance for prepartum dairy cows with specific reference to hypocalcemic parturient paresis. Can J Anim Sci 1989;69:411–7.

27. Goff JP, Horst RL, Mueller FJ, et al. Addition of chloride to a prepartal diet high in cations increases 1,25-dihydroxyvitamin D response to hypocalcemia preventing milk fever. J Dairy Sci 1991;74(11):3863–71.

28. Phillippo M, Reid GW, Nevison IM. Parturient hypocalcaemia in dairy cows: effects of dietary acidity on plasma minerals and calciotrophic hormones. Res Vet Sci 1994;56(3):303–9.

29. Abu Damir H, Phillippo M, Thorp BH, et al. Effects of dietary acidity on calcium balance and mobilisation, bone morphology and 1,25- dihydroxyvitamin D in prepartal dairy cows. Res Vet Sci 1994;56:310–8.

30. Liesegang A. Influence of anionic salts on bone metabolism in periparturient dairy goats and sheep. J Dairy Sci 2008;91(6):2449–60.

31. van Mosel M, Wouterse HS, van't Klooster AT. Effects of reducing dietary ([Na+ + K+]-[Cl- + SO4 =]) on bone in dairy cows at parturition. Res Vet Sci 1994;56(3):270–6.

32. Schonewille JT, Van't Klooster AT, Wouterse H, et al. Hypocalcemia induced by intravenous administration of disodium ethylenediaminotetraacetate and its effects on excretion of calcium in urine of cows fed a high chloride diet. J Dairy Sci 1999;82(6):1317–24.

33. Batlle D, Itsarayoungyuen K, Hays S, et al. Parathyroid hormone is not anticalciuric during chronic metabolic acidosis. Kidney Int 1982;22(3):264–71.

34. Lemann J Jr, Bushinsky DA, Hamm LL. Bone buffering of acid and base in humans. Am J Physiol Renal Physiol 2003;285(5):F811–32.

35. Vagg MJ, Payne JM. The effect of ammonium chloride induced acidosis on calcium metabolism in ruminants. Br Vet J 1970;126(10):531–7.

36. Braithwaite GD. The effect of ammonium chloride on calcium metabolism in sheep. Br J Nutr 1972;27(1):201–9.

37. Wang C, Beede DK. Effects of ammonium chloride and sulfate on acid-base status and calcium metabolism of dry Jersey cows. J Dairy Sci 1992;75(3):820–8.

38. Tucker WB, Hogue JF, Waterman DF, et al. Role of sulfur and chloride in the dietary cation-anion balance equation for lactating dairy cattle. J Anim Sci 1991; 69(3):1205–13.

39. Oetzel GR, Fettman MJ, Hamar DW, et al. Screening of anionic salts for palatability, effects on acid-base status, and urinary calcium excretion in dairy cows. J Dairy Sci 1991;74(3):965–71.

40. Goff JP, Ruiz R, Horst RL. Relative acidifying activity of anionic salts commonly used to prevent milk fever. J Dairy Sci 2004;87(5):1245–55.

41. Constable PD. Clinical assessment of acid-base status. Strong ion difference theory. Vet Clin North Am Food Anim Pract 1999;15(3):447–71.

42. Beede DK, Pilbeam TE, Puffenbarger SM, et al. Peripartum responses of Holstein cows and heifers fed graded concentrations of calcium (calcium carbonate) and anion (chloride) three weeks before calving [abstract]. J Dairy Sci 2001;84:83.

43. Peterson AB, Orth MW, Goff JP, et al. Periparturient responses of multiparous Holstein cows fed different dietary phosphorus concentrations prepartum. J Dairy Sci 2005;88(10):3582–94.

44. Barton BA, Jorgensen NA, DeLuca HF. Impact of prepartum dietary phosphorus intake on calcium homeostasis at parturition. J Dairy Sci 1987;70(6):1186–91.

45. Kichura TS, Horst RL, Beitz DC, et al. Relationships between prepartal dietary calcium and phosphorus, vitamin D metabolism, and parturient paresis in dairy cows. J Nutr 1982;112(3):480–7.

46. Cheng Y, Goff JP, Horst RL. Restoring normal blood phosphorus concentrations in hypophosphatemic cattle with sodium phosphate. Vet Med 1998;93:383–6.

47. Gould DH, McAllister MM, Savage JC, et al. High sulfide concentrations in rumen fluid associated with nutritionally induced polioencephalomalacia in calves. Am J Vet Res 1991;52(7):1164–9.

48. Jardon P. Using urine pH to monitor anionic salt programs. Compend Contin Educ Pract Vet 1995;17:860–2.

49. Thomas ED. What we're learning about growing grasses for dry cows. Hoard's Dairyman 1996;141:224.
50. Pelletier S, Tremblay GF, Bélanger G, et al. Nutritive value of timothy fertilized with chloride or chloride-containing liquid swine manure. J Dairy Sci 2008; 91(2):713–21.
51. Goff JP, Brummer EC, Henning SJ, et al. Effect of application of ammonium chloride and calcium chloride on alfalfa cation-anion content and yield. J Dairy Sci 2007;90(11):5159–64.
52. van Mosel M, van't Klooster AT, Wouterse HS. Effects of a deficient magnesium supply during the dry period on bone turnover of dairy cows at parturition. Vet Q 1991;13(4):199–208.
53. DeGaris PJ, Lean IJ. Milk fever in dairy cows: a review of pathophysiology and control principles. Vet J 2008;176(1):58–69.
54. Resnick LM, Altura BT, Gupta RK, et al. Intracellular and extracellular magnesium depletion in type 2 (non-insulin-dependent) diabetes mellitus. Diabetologia 1993;36(8):767–70.
55. Rude RK. Magnesium deficiency: a cause of heterogeneous disease in humans. J Bone Miner Res 1998;13(4):749–58.
56. van de Braak AE, van't Klooster AT, Malestein A. Influence of a deficient supply of magnesium during the dry period on the rate of calcium mobilisation by dairy cows at parturition. Res Vet Sci 1987;42(1):101–8.
57. Rude RK, Oldham SB, Sharp CF Jr, et al. Parathyroid hormone secretion in magnesium deficiency. J Clin Endocrinol Metab 1978;47(4):800–6.
58. Fatemi S, Ryzen E, Flores J, et al. Effect of experimental human magnesium depletion on parathyroid hormone secretion and 1,25-dihydroxyvitamin D metabolism. J Clin Endocrinol Metab 1991;73:1067–72.
59. Littledike ET, Stuedemann JA, Wilkinson SR, et al. Grass tetany syndrome. Role of magnesium in animal nutrition. Blacksburg (VA): Virginia Polytechnic Inst. and State Univ; 1983. p. 173.
60. Goings RL, Jacobson NL, Beitz DC, et al. Prevention of parturient paresis by a prepartum, calcium-deficient diet. J Dairy Sci 1974;57(10):1184–8.
61. Green HB, Horst RL, Beitz DC, et al. Vitamin D metabolites in plasma of cows fed a prepartum low-calcium diet for prevention of parturient hypocalcemia. J Dairy Sci 1981;64(2):217–26.
62. Thilsing-Hansen T, Jorgensen RJ, Enemark JM, et al. The effect of zeolite A supplementation in the dry period on periparturient calcium, phosphorus, and magnesium homeostasis. J Dairy Sci 2002;85(7):1855–62.
63. Hibbs JW, Conrad HR. Milk fever in dairy cows. VII. Effect of continuous vitamin D feeding on incidence of milk fever. J Dairy Sci 1976;59(11):1944–6.
64. Littledike ET, Horst RL. Problems with vitamin D injections for prevention of milk fever: toxicity of large doses and increased incidence of small doses. J Dairy Sci 1979;63:89.
65. Bar A, Perlman R, Sachs M. Observation on the use of 1 alpha-hydroxyvitamin D3 in the prevention of bovine parturient paresis: the effect of a single injection on plasma 1 alpha-hydroxyvitamin D3, 1,25-dihydroxyvitamin D3, calcium, and hydroxyproline. J Dairy Sci 1985;68(8):1952–8.
66. Hove K, Kristiansen T. Oral 1,25-dihydroxyvitamin D3 in prevention of milk fever. Acta Vet Scand 1984;25(4):510–25.
67. Goff JP, Horst RL. Effect of subcutaneously released 24F-1,25-dihydroxyvitamin D3 on incidence of parturient paresis in dairy cows. J Dairy Sci 1990;73(2): 406–12.

68. Goff JP. Treatment of calcium, phosphorus, and magnesium balance disorders. Vet Clin North Am Food Anim Pract 1999;15(3):619–39.

69. Pehrson B, Svensson C, Jonsson M. A comparative study of the effectiveness of calcium propionate and calcium chloride for the prevention of parturient paresis in dairy cows. J Dairy Sci 1998;81:2011–6.

70. Goff JP, Brown TR, Stokes SR, et al. Titration of the proper dose of calcium propionate (NutroCAL) to be included in an oral drench for fresh cows. J Dairy Sci 2002;85(Suppl 1):189.

71. Melendez P, Donovan A, Risco CA, et al. Metabolic responses of transition Holstein cows fed anionic salts and supplemented at calving with calcium and energy. J Dairy Sci 2002;85(5):1085–92.

72. Goff JP, Horst RL. Oral administration of calcium salts for treatment of hypocalcemia in cattle. J Dairy Sci 1993;76:101–8.

73. Horst RL, Goff JP, Reinhardt TA. Advancing age results in reduction of intestinal and bone 1,25-dihydroxyvitamin D receptor. Endocrinology 1990;126(2): 1053–7.

74. Hanai H, Brennan DP, Cheng L, et al. Down regulation of parathyroid hormone receptors in renal membranes from aged rats. Am J Physiol 1990;259(3 Pt 2): F444–50.

75. Goff JP, Reinhardt TA, Beitz DB, et al. Breed affects tissue vitamin D receptor concentration in periparturient dairy cows: a milk fever risk factor? [abstract]. J Dairy Sci 1995;78(Suppl 1):184.

76. Liesegang A, Singer K, Boos A. Vitamin D receptor amounts across different segments of the gastrointestinal tract in Brown Swiss and Holstein Friesian cows of different age. J Anim Physiol Anim Nutr 2008;92:316–23.

77. Mayland H. Grass tetany. In: Church D, editor. The ruminant animal: digestive physiology and nutrition. Prospect Heights (IL): Waveland Press, Inc; 1988. p. 511–23.

78. Martens H, Gabel G. Pathogenesis and prevention of grass tetany from the physiologic viewpoint. Dtsch Tierarztl Wochenschr 1986;93:170 [in German].

79. Martens H, Rayssiguier Y. Magnesium metabolism and hypomagnesemia. In: Ruckebusch Y, Thivend P, editors. Digestive physiology and metabolism in ruminants. Lancaster (England): MTP Press; 1980. p. 447–66.

80. Pfeffer E, Thompson A, Armstrong DG. Studies on intestinal digestion in the sheep. 3. Net movement of certain inorganic elements in the digestive tract on rations containing different proportions of hay and rolled barley. Br J Nutr 1970;24(1):197–204.

81. Care AD, Brown RC, Farrar AR, et al. Magnesium absorption from the digestive tract of sheep. Q J Exp Physiol 1984;69(3):577–87.

82. Greene LW, Fontenot JP, Webb KE Jr. Site of magnesium and other macromineral absorption in steers fed high levels of potassium. J Anim Sci 1983;57(2): 503–10.

83. Martens H, Schweigel M. Pathophysiology of grass tetany and other hypomagnesemias. Implications for clinical management. Vet Clin North Am Food Anim Pract 2000;16(2):339–68.

84. Cook GM, Wells JE, Russell JB. Ability of Acidaminococcus fermentans to oxidize trans-aconitate and decrease the accumulation of tricarballylate, a toxic end product of ruminal fermentation. Appl Environ Microbiol 1994;60(7):2533–7.

85. Ram L, Schonewille JT, Martens H, et al. Magnesium absorption by wethers fed potassium bicarbonate in combination with different dietary magnesium concentrations. J Dairy Sci 1998;81(9):2485–92.

86. Newton GL, Fontenot JP, Tucker RE, et al. Effects of high dietary potassium intake on the metabolism of magnesium by sheep. J Anim Sci 1972;35(2):440–5.
87. Jittakhot S, Schonewille JT, Wouterse H, et al. Increasing magnesium intakes in relation to magnesium absorption in dry cows. J Dairy Res 2004;71(3):297–303.
88. Schonewille JT, van't Klooster AT, van Mosel M. A comparative study of the in-vitro solubility and availability of magnesium from various sources for cattle. Tijdschr Diergeneeskd 1992;117(4):105–8 [in Dutch].

Treatment of Phosphorus Balance Disorders

Walter Grünberg, Dr med vet, MS, PhD

KEYWORDS

- Hypophosphatemia • Phosphorus • Homeostasis • Cattle • Treatment

KEY POINTS

- With phosphorus (P) a predominantly intracellular electrolyte, accurately assessing the P status of an individual animal remains a challenge.
- The P concentration in serum or plasma, although widely used to diagnose P balance disorders, is an unreliable parameter for this purpose.
- In many instances, the causative relation between acute hypophosphatemia and the clinical signs associated with it are not well established.
- Organic P compounds contained in pharmaceutical products intended for parenteral treatment in food-producing animals often provide P in a form that is not effectively converted into phosphate (PO_4). These compounds are, therefore, unsuitable for P supplementation.
- Intravenous (IV) bolus infusion of sodium PO_4 salt solutions has an immediate but very short-lived effect on the serum P concentration.
- Oral supplementation of PO_4 salts presents a practical and effective treatment alternative in P-depleted animals but seems to require some degree of rumen motility.

FUNCTIONS OF PHOSPHORUS IN THE ORGANISM

P is an essential macromineral with a plethora of important biologic functions. P plays a structural role at tissue, cellular, and molecular levels of any living organism. P in bone and teeth provides these tissues with their characteristic rigidity and stability. Cellular integrity depends on P that forms an integral part of the phospholipids that form cell membranes. P is also incorporated in nucleic acid molecules, such as DNA and RNA. The regulation of metabolism on a cellular level is highly dependent on the availability of P for phosphorylation, a chemical reaction where P is added to an enzyme or other molecule, thereby modulating the biologic activity of this molecule. Energy is transported and stored within cells in the form of high-energy PO_4 bonds,

Conflict of interest disclosure: The author has no conflicts of interest to report.
Clinic for Cattle, University of Veterinary Medicine Hannover, Foundation, Bischofsholer Damm 15, 30173 Hanover, Germany
E-mail address: waltergruenberg@yahoo.com

Vet Clin Food Anim 30 (2014) 383–408
http://dx.doi.org/10.1016/j.cvfa.2014.03.002   vetfood.theclinics.com

such as ATP or creatine PO_4. PO_4 is an effective buffer in biologic fluids, such as cytosol, urine, or rumen fluid, thereby contributing to maintaining the acid-base equilibrium in the organism. By being the quantitatively most important intracellular anion, P is a major contributor to the transmembrane potential and the osmotic equilibrium between intra- and extracellular space.[1–3] In ruminants, P is an essential nutrient for ruminal microorganisms where it is required for the fermentation of cellulose and the synthesis of microbial protein.[4–6]

Phosphorus, Inorganic Phosphorus, and Phosphate

Elemental P is highly reactive and too unstable to occur as such in nature. The most commonly encountered form of P is PO_4, that is, the maximally oxidized form of P. In the body, P is present as PO_4 that is either unbound and, therefore, also called inorganic P or orthophosphate (Pi), or chemically bonded to a carbon-containing molecule, in which case it is referred to it as either organic P or organic PO_4 (Po). It is, therefore, tempting to use the terms, P and PO_4, interchangeably but, strictly speaking, Pi is the P contained in inorganic PO_4, whereas inorganic PO_4 refers to the entire unbound PO_4 molecule. Differentiating between P and PO_4 is important when concentrations of Pi are expressed on a weight rather than a molar basis (ie, in mg/dL instead of mmol/L). Whereas 1 mol of P is equivalent to 1 mol of PO_4, the masses of the atom P and the molecule PO_4 are different. The widely accepted reference range of the serum Pi concentration [Pi] is 1.4 to 2.6 mmol/L, which is equivalent to 4.0 to 8.0 mg/dL of Pi but 12.3 to 24.7 mg/dL of inorganic PO_4.[3] The reference range of 4.0 to 8.0 mg/dL thus refers to the concentration of [P] and not of PO_4.

Inorganic PO_4 in the body is present either in its divalent (HPO_4^{2-}) or its monovalent form ($H_2PO_4^-$), with the ratio $HPO_4^{2-}:H_2PO_4^-$ depending on the ambient pH. At a pH of 7.4, this ratio is approximately 4:1 but decreases with decreasing pH. The divalent form can be considered an effective buffer that is able to bind 1 H^+, whereas the monovalent form can be considered a used buffer that does not bind any more protons at the pH range normally encountered in the body.

The ammonium molybdate method is the standard clinical chemistry procedure used to determine [P] in body fluids, such as serum, plasma, whole blood, urine, or saliva, and is based on a reaction of molybdate with the PO_4 molecule to form a phosphomolybdate complex. This method specifically measures the [Pi] rather than the [P]. In contrast, P in tissue, feed, feces, or milk is generally measured using methods determining the total P content.

For phosphorylation and the synthesis of any P-containing organic molecule, the organism requires the availability of inorganic PO_4, which is the only known substrate that can be used for phosphorylation. To effectively supplement an animal with P, therefore, requires providing either inorganic PO_4 or a P-containing compound that can be readily hydrolyzed in the organism to release the inorganic PO_4.

In this article, P refers to P contained in either organic or inorganic PO_4, whereas Pi refers to P contained in inorganic PO_4 alone.

Distribution of Phosphorus in the Body

In vertebrates, 80% to 85% of the body's P is located in the skeleton, primarily in the form of insoluble salts, namely calcium phosphate ($Ca_3[PO_4]_2$) and dihydroxyapatite ($Ca_{10}[PO_4]_6[OH]_2$), which present the biologically inert storage form of P. Between 15% and 20% of the body P is distributed in fluids and soft tissues of the body, thus forming the body P pool.

The bulk of the body P pool is located in the intracellular space, whereas less than 1% of the total body P content is found in the extracellular space. The intracellular [P] has been estimated to be approximately 100 mmol/L, of which the largest part is incorporated in organic compounds, such as adenosine PO_4, NADP, or phosphorylated carbohydrate metabolites. In comparison, the Pi fraction in the intracellular space is minute, with intracellular [Pi] in the range of 1 mmol/L, which is below the extracellular [Pi].[7] To complicate matters, the intracellular space cannot be considered a single compartment for P distribution. Within the cell, different organelles, such as cytosolic mitochondria, are able to sequester Pi to meet their metabolic P requirements and thus present separate intracellular compartments with different [Pi].[8]

The extracellular P pool can be subdivided into 2 large fractions that include the P bound in lipoprotein molecules and the Pi fraction. The concentration of P bound in lipoproteins is above 1.8 mmol/L (>5 mg/dL) P in adult cattle, whereas the [Pi] is approximately 1.5 mmol/L.[9-11] Approximately 10% of the extracellular Pi fraction is bound to protein and another 5% is complexed to cations, such as calcium (Ca) and magnesium (Mg). Plasma is part of the extracellular space and accordingly the concentration of [Pi] in serum or plasma is considered a valid surrogate parameter for the extracellular [Pi].

PHOSPHORUS HOMEOSTASIS AND HOMEORHESIS

P homeostasis refers to the equilibrium of the bioavailable P pool, which includes intra- and extracellular P but not the metabolically inert P fraction stored in bones. The organism's P balance is dictated by the equilibrium between uptake and excretion of P to which the exchange of P between bone and extracellular space as well as between intra- and extracellular space has to be added (**Fig. 1**).[12] Uptake of P exclusively occurs through the gastrointestinal tract from where P is absorbed and then transferred to the extracellular space for further distribution throughout the body. Absorbed P may be retained and transferred into bone or the intracellular space of different tissues or excreted from the organism.

Excretion of P in monogastric species primarily occurs through the kidneys. In ruminants, in contrast, under physiologic conditions, renal excretion of P in quantitatively relevant amounts only occurs in preruminating young animals as well as in nonlactating ruminants fed a high-concentrate diet with high P content. Feces and milk (in lactating cows) present the most important routes of P excretion in ruminants.[13] Fecal

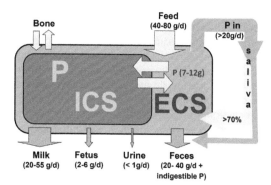

Fig. 1. P homeorhesis of a lactating dairy cow (600 kg). The outer rectangle represents the extracellular space (ECS); the inner rectangle represents the intracellular space (ICS). P represents the total P content of the intracellular and extracellular space; numbers in parenthesis give the amount of P in grams.

P consists of unabsorbed dietary P and endogenously lost P as well as unreabsorbed salivary P. Excretion of P in saliva is a peculiarity of ruminants that assures adequate P supply to ruminal microorganisms and provides a buffer to rumen fluid. The [Pi] in ruminant saliva ranges between 4 and 15 mmol/L (12–46 mg/dL), which is considerably above the [Pi] of serum. Assuming a daily saliva production of approximately 230 L in adult lactating cows, salivary P excretion can be estimated to range between 25 and 100 g of P per day. Salivary P is reabsorbed from the intestinal tract with at least the same efficiency as dietary P (approximately 80%).[3,14,15] P excreted through saliva is thus not lost but just transiently unavailable to the organism. The unabsorbed fraction of salivary P contributes the fecal P content.

In high-yielding dairy cows, the mammary gland contributes considerably to daily P losses. P concentrations in bovine milk range between 0.7 and 1.3 g/L.[16–18] The [P] of colostrum is higher than that of milk but declines within the first week of lactation. Daily P losses through the mammary gland can thus easily exceed 40 g in high-yielding dairy cows. This P drain presents a considerable challenge to the mechanisms regulating P homeostasis, particularly at the onset of lactation. The ruminant mammary gland maintains constant concentrations of minerals, such as Ca and P in milk, independently of the availability of these elements to the maternal organism to assure adequate mineral supply to the calf.[19,20] Losses of P through the mammary gland can, therefore, only be reduced by decreasing milk production.

Maternal losses of P related to pregnancy are considered negligible in the first 2 trimesters of pregnancy. During the last trimester, the daily rate of P accretion in the bovine fetus increases from 1.9 g/d at 190 days to 5.4 g/d at 280 days of gestation.[21]

Exchanges of P between bone and the P pool are balanced and quantitatively near nil in adult animals with adequate P supply. Growing animals have a net flux of P toward bone to assure adequate mineralization of the bone matrix whereas older and P-depleted animals tend to have a net flux of P from bone to the P pool.[22] Acidogenic diets trigger the demineralization of the bone matrix, thereby releasing Ca and Pi. Long-standing metabolic acidosis therefore results in a net flux of P together with Ca from bone to the P pool.[23]

The equilibrium between intra- and extracellular space is a major factor affecting the extracellular [Pi] and thus the serum [Pi]. The regulation and pathway of P transport in and out of the cells are still poorly understood. Although cell membranes are sufficiently permeable to Pi to allow a detectable bulk movement of Pi across cell membranes, active or facilitated transport mechanisms are essential to assure adequate Pi supply to the intracellular space. Most of the currently known Pi transport pathways are coupled to sodium transport and take advantage of the sodium gradient between intra- and extracellular space.[24,25] Changes in the equilibrium of Pi between intra- and extracellular space can occur suddenly and have a considerable impact on the extracellular [Pi]. Factors affecting the compartmental redistribution of Pi are, among others, the insulin and catecholamine secretion of the body or the acid-base status of the organism.[12,26] An increase in plasma insulin concentration, as observed after feeding or parenteral dextrose administration, increases the uptake of Pi by insulin responsive cells, thereby resulting in a decrease of the extracellular [Pi].[27,28]

Acidemia and metabolic acidosis decrease the cellular Pi uptake presumably by impairing the glycolytic pathway.[26] In contrast, metabolic, and, particularly, respiratory alkalosis enhance cellular Pi uptake, thereby causing a decline in serum [Pi].[26]

Surges in the blood catecholamine concentration have been associated with marked declines in serum [Pi], an effect that is at least in part believed attributable to an intracellular Pi shift.[29]

Regulation of Phosphorus Homeostasis

The regulation of the P homeostasis in ruminants and other species is still not entirely understood. Several endocrine substances, such as parathyroid hormone (PTH), vitamin D_3, calcitonin, insulin, and cathecholamines, are known to affect P homeostasis in mammals. None of these hormones seems to regulate the P homeostasis in direct response to changes of the extracellular [Pi] because no sensors for the extracellular Pi concentrations have been identified.[22]

PTH can increase P excretion through urine and saliva and trigger mobilization of Pi from bone, thus having a strong impact on the body's P homeostasis. Notwithstanding, renal tubular cells and bovine salivary gland cells become unresponsive to PTH in states of severe P depletion, which suggests that intrinsic regulation at the cellular level can overrule the effect of PTH in case of severe P depletion.[30,31] This overrule switch in states of marked deregulation of the P homeostasis questions the concept of PTH functioning as an effective regulator of the P homeostasis.

Vitamin D_3 is known to enhance intestinal P absorption and to control PTH secretion through a negative feedback mechanism.[22] Studies in ruminants and other species revealed that intestinal P absorption can be up-regulated in states of P deficiency independently of vitamin D_3, again suggesting the presence of an alternative regulatory circuit of intestinal P uptake.[32,33] Intrinsic regulation of sodium dependent Pi uptake has thus far been demonstrated for renal tubular cells, liver cells, heart muscle cells, osteoblasts, and epithelial cells of the proximal small intestine.[33–35]

Insulin strongly affects the equilibrium between intra- and extracellular space by triggering a quantitatively important intracellular P shift, presumably to satisfy increased requirements resulting from increased carbohydrate metabolism.

Endogenous as well as parenterally administered epinephrine decreases the serum [Pi] in humans and other species. Although a β-adrenergic stimulation of cellular Pi uptake is considered the primary mechanism in humans, in cattle, cathecholamines were found to also trigger a release of PTH.[29,36] Although the effect of catecholamines on the P homeostasis in cattle does not seem to have been studied, it is conceivable that increased PTH secretion enhances renal and salivary Pi excretion in ruminants.

Calcitonin, a polypeptide synthesized in the parathyroid gland, is among the endocrine substances considered relevant for the equilibrium of extracellular Ca and Pi. The role of calcitonin, whose primary function is to prevent hypercalcemia in the extracellular space, was found essential for aquatic organisms living in a high-Ca environment. The importance of calcitonin for the regulation of Ca and P homeostasis in mammals in contrast is under contentious debate.[37]

Phosphatonins are a novel group of substances influencing the P homeostasis specifically by modulating renal tubular reabsorption of P as well as inhibiting activation of vitamin D_3.[38] The precise mechanism through which the synthesis of phosphatonins is regulated is not yet understood and the role of phosphatonis in ruminants has not yet been studied.

Assessment of Phosphorus Status

Although P deficiency in ruminants and other species is widespread, a satisfactory method to objectively assess the P status of an individual animal is still not available. Several parameters have been proposed over the years, such as [Pi] in plasma or serum, saliva, red blood cells or whole blood, urine, rumen fluid, feces, or the content of P in bone and other tissues.

Phosphorus concentration in serum or plasma

Serum [Pi] and plasma [Pi] are the most commonly used parameters to assess the P status of an individual animal. In general, the serum [Pi] correlates well with the short-term dietary P supply and the P pool size, would there not be substantial and sudden fluctuations of the serum [Pi] that are independent of changes in P intake or P pool size. Factors causing such fluctuations of the serum [Pi] are discussed later. In contrast, the serum [Pi] poorly reflects states and degree of chronic P deficiency because mobilization of P reserves from bone compensates for long-standing inadequate P supply, thereby masking P depletion at least partially.[39–41]

Phosphorus concentration in whole blood or in red blood cells

The whole blood [Pi] that is measured in blood after inducing complete hemolysis was proposed as a more accurate parameter to estimate the total P pool size because it contains intra- and extracellular Pi.[39,42] Because the [Pi] in whole blood strongly depends on the blood packed cell volume, which can vary considerably between animals independently of the P status, this parameter is unlikely to reliably reflect the P status of an animal.

Alternatively, the [Pi] in red blood cells has been suggested as parameter to estimate the [Pi] in intracellular fluid.[42] A potential issue arises from the use of the ammonium molybdate method that is the standard analytical procedure in clinical chemistry, specifically measuring [Pi]. With the ongoing and rapid release of [Pi] during the decay of organic compounds, such as ATP, sample handling and, most of all, time from collection to analysis are likely to have a great impact on the analysis.[43] Furthermore, it remains to be determined to what degree the erythrocytes are actually representative of the body's average intracellular Pi pool.[8]

Phosphorus concentration in saliva

The association between dietary P intake and saliva [Pi] and between serum and saliva [Pi] has been studied extensively in ruminants.[44–46] Although the effects of altering dietary P content on the salivary [Pi] over time within one animal is well documented, there is little evidence of any close relationship between salivary [Pi] in dietary P content between animals.[46] Several factors complicate the interpretation of saliva [Pi]. The [Pi] in saliva varies markedly between salivary glands. With the salivary flow of different glands variable over time, the composition of a saliva sample and thus its [Pi] is likely to vary as well.[44] Furthermore, it was found that salivary [Pi] was maintained at disproportionately high levels as dietary P intake decreases in the short term.[47] Finally, to assure that saliva samples have been neither contaminated with feed particles nor diluted by drinking water, measuring other parameters, such as salivary osmolality or sodium concentration, is necessary, which adds to the costs of this diagnostic approach. The salivary [Pi] was deemed less reliable than serum [Pi] to estimate the daily P supply or the P status of an animal.[45]

Phosphorus concentration in urine

Although urine is the primary route of P excretion in monogastric species, the amount of P excreted through the kidney in healthy ruminants is negligible. Reported values for renal P excretion in dairy cows vary considerably but generally are below 1% of the dietary P intake, and [Pi] in urine of adult ruminants are often around or below the detection limit of the standard biochemical assays.[23,48,49] Furthermore, renal Pi handling is strongly influenced by the Ca homeostasis, PTH secretion, and the urine pH. Aciduria as well as hypocalcemia and ensuing increased PTH secretion both can result in increased renal Pi excretion that is independent of the body's P status.[48,50] Because there is no clear relationship between renal Pi excretion and the

P status of the body, neither the urinary [Pi] nor any derived parameter, such as the fractional Pi excretion or the Pi-to-creatinine ratio in urine, can be considered reliable surrogate parameters for the Pi status in adult ruminants.

Phosphorus concentration in feces or rumen fluid

The association between dietary P intake and the concentrations of P in fecal or rumen fluid samples has been explored in several studies. Although the effect of the dietary P content on the intestinal absorption rate of P is well established, neither rumen fluid samples nor fecal grab samples were found to reliably identify P-depleted animals. Specifically, when P-depleted animals show feed intake depression, a clinical sign often associated with P deficiency, fecal output decreases. This can translate into unchanged or even increased fecal [P] although the total fecal P output is decreased.[51]

The rumen fluid [Pi] in contrast is a function of the dietary P content, feed intake, saliva production, and rumen motility. Decreasing the dietary P supply in ruminants was shown to result in an initial decline in rumen fluid [Pi] that rapidly reached a plateau despite ongoing P losses.[41] Apparently, the previously described up-regulation of the salivary P excretion in states of P depletion prevents an excessive decline of the [Pi] in rumen fluid, thereby rendering the rumen fluid [Pi] unsuitable to assess the P status in ruminants.[40,47]

Bone phosphorus content

The P content in fresh bone was found a reliable criterion to assess body P reserves but it is considered less suitable to assess current dietary P supply or the body P pool size.[40,52] The body responds to chronic P depletion by mobilizing minerals from the bone matrix and then replenishes bone stores after the deficiency has been corrected. Nonetheless, the bone P content is slow to respond to changes in dietary P supply, which means that the nutritional history has a strong impact on the mineral content of fresh bone. The P content in fresh bone is, therefore, an excellent indicator for the body P reserves but not for the current dietary P supply or the P pool size.[52,53] Because obtaining bone biopsies is impractical under field conditions, determination of bone P content is largely restricted to postmortem examination or research.

Soft tissue phosphorus content

Soft tissue, more specifically, muscle tissue, has been proposed as the most relevant specimen to assess the P status of the organism because it is quantitatively among the most important tissues and because many of the clinical signs associated with P depletion are associated with effects on muscle tissue.[8,54,55] Dietary P depletion over a course of several weeks was associated with a decline in striated muscle tissue P content in different mammal species that was less pronounced than the concomitant decline observed in serum [Pi].[55–57] Serum [Pi] and muscle tissue P content were found correlated in a nonlinear manner.[55,57] Few studies exploring the effect of P depletion on soft tissue P content have been conducted in ruminants. Tissue samples of heart, muscle, kidney, and liver from heifers fed diets that were either deficient or adequate in P content for more than 1 year did not differ in their total P content.[40] The apparent discrepancy between this and the previously discussed studies could be due to the different duration of dietary P depletion. Long-standing P deficiency results in P mobilization from bone to prevent an excessive decline of the total P pool size and thereby the P content in muscle tissue.

Serum Phosphorus Concentration

Despite the difficult interpretation of the [Pi] in serum or plasma, this parameter is still the most commonly used measurement for the P status in human and veterinary medicine. With plasma forming part of the extracellular space, the serum or plasma [Pi] is widely accepted as valid surrogate parameter for the [Pi] in extracellular fluid. Reference ranges for cattle given in the literature are 1.4 to 2.6 mmol/L (4.0–8.0 mg/dL) and 1.9 to 2.6 mmol/L (6.0–8.0 mg/dL) for adult and growing animals, respectively.[3] The reference range for sheep and goats is 1.6 to 2.4 mmol/L (5.0–7.3 mg/dL) and 1.3 to 3.0 mmol/L (4.2–9.1 mg/dL), respectively.[58] Juvenile and growing individuals have higher serum [Pi] due to enhanced intestinal Pi uptake presumably to provide sufficient Pi for adequate bone mineralization.[59,60]

Several factors around blood sample collection can have an effect on the [Pi] of the analyzed sample and should be taken into consideration when interpreting the laboratory results.

Site of blood sample collection

The serum [Pi] can vary depending on the vessel from which blood is collected. Serum [Pi] obtained from the coccygeal vein or artery blood ranges between 4% and 19% above concentrations determined in serum from jugular venous blood.[61–64] This considerable difference was attributed to the substantial P drain through salivary glands, thereby lowering the [Pi] in jugular blood. Serum [Pi] measured in blood from the udder vein was found in the same range of the serum [Pi] of coccygeal vein blood.[63]

Anticoagulants

Plasma [Pi] was found slightly lower than serum [Pi], but differences were below 5% and thus considered of little practical relevance. The difference has been attributed to ongoing hydrolysis of organic P compounds releasing Pi in blood samples collected in serum tubes that have to sit to allow clotting before being centrifuged.[40,64]

Using tubes containing sodium fluoride as anticoagulant yields [Pi] 10% below concentrations measured in sodium heparin plasma or serum.[63] This effect has been explained with the marked increase of the osmolality of the blood sample in sodium fluoride tubes that causes a shift of cell water to the extracellular space, thereby diluting plasma.[43]

Sample collection and sample processing

Poor blood collection technique resulting in hemolysis results in release of intracellular Pi and thereby falsely increases the measured plasma [Pi]. Furthermore, separation of serum or plasma from blood cells should be done within 4 hours of collection, taking care to prevent hemolysis. Delayed harvesting of serum or plasma results in elevated [Pi] from ongoing hydrolysis of organic P compounds as well as from erythrolysis.[43]

Presample collection factors

Other factors potentially affecting the serum [Pi], such as sampling time relative to feed intake, water intake, or time of the day, have been studied but results are inconsistent.[40,64,65]

Physical exercise (eg, repeated unsuccessful attempts to get up) or treatment with IV dextrose within 2 to 3 hours before blood sampling can result in artifactually decreased serum [Pi] with a difference in the range of 20% and above. These changes are largely due to sudden redistribution of P between intra- and extracellular space (discussed later).[28,65]

HYPOPHOSPHATEMIA
Mechanisms of Hypophosphatemia

Hypophosphatemia refers to a decline of the serum [Pi] below the established reference range and can be the result of inadequate dietary P supply, excessive losses of P (through milk, feces, or urine), a compartmental shift of P from the extracellular into the intracellular space, or a combination of 2 or all of these mechanisms. Although the first 2 mechanisms are consistent with P depletion of the organism, a compartmental shift of P to the intracellular space results in hypophosphatemia without a concomitant reduction of the total P pool size (**Fig. 2**). It is, therefore, important to consider different etiologic scenarios when interpreting subnormal serum [Pi].

Hypophosphatemia due to inadequate dietary P supply

P depletion due to either anorexia or consumption of diets with inadequate P content can result in P depletion within days and in general is associated with a decline in serum [Pi].[12,66] Although animals grazing on P-deficient soils suffer from chronic P depletion, individuals going off feed for several days develop a depletion of the P pool and hypophosphatemia more acutely.[53,66] Hypophosphatemia is a common finding in cattle that have been off feed for several days.[66,67]

Hypophosphatemia due to excessive P losses

An example of hypophosphatemia resulting from excessive P excretion is hypophosphatemia in fresh cows that is at least in part caused by the sudden increase of P requirements for milk production at the onset of lactation.[68] Another common cause of increased P losses is aciduria that can be observed in ruminants on an acidogenic diets or in sick individuals.[50,67] In cattle with acidic urine, renal tubular Pi reabsorption is markedly decreased, presumably with the goal of providing an additional buffer for urine.[50] Other less common causes for excessive P losses include renal disorders, such as Fanconi syndrome or the primary hyperparathyroidism.

Hypophosphatemia due to compartmental P shifts

As discussed previously, sudden redistribution of P between intra- and extracellular space occurs frequently and can have a marked impact on the serum [Pi]. Mechanisms regulating the equilibrium of P between intra- and extracellular space are still poorly understood. Apart from passive diffusion of P across cell membranes along a chemical gradient, cells can modulate P uptake by activating specific transport mechanisms to meet their metabolic requirements.[8] The classic example of such a mechanism is the intracellular shift of P that is triggered by insulin.[27,28] Parenteral administration of dextrose either as bolus or drip at a dose commonly used in practice lowers the plasma [Pi] within minutes by more than 30%.

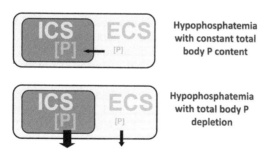

Fig. 2. Different types of hypophosphatemia that cannot be differentiated based on the plasma PO_4 concentration. The upper panel shows hypophosphatemia caused by a compartmental shift of P toward the intracellular space whereas the total body P content remains unchanged. The lower panel shows hypophosphatemia due to a loss of total body P (decline of intracellular and extracellular PO_4). ECS, extracellular space; ICS, intracellular space; [P], phosphorus concentration.

A deregulation of the acid-base equilibrium can also affect the P equilibrium between intra- and extracellular space, with acidemia inhibiting and alkalemia (in particular respiratory alkalosis) enhancing cellular Pi uptake.[26] This effect has been attributed to impaired insulin sensitivity in states of acidosis or acidemia.[69,70] Decreased insulin response to a glucose load and possibly also insulin sensitivity have been documented in acidotic cattle and other mammalian species.[26,71]

Hypophosphatemia due to a combination of several mechanisms

Hypophosphatemia in periparturient cattle is a common finding with multifactorial etiology. The sudden onset of milk production draining approximately 1 g of P for every kilogram of milk produced is without doubt an important contributing factor to the deregulation of the P homeostasis around calving. The decline in dry matter intake observed in the last week before calving is likely to contribute to hypophosphatemia around parturition or at least to hamper counter-regulation. A marked drop in serum [Pi] around calving is also observed in mastectomized cows not producing any milk.[72,73] This observation underscores that factors other than milk production must be involved in the etiology of periparturient hypophosphatemia of dairy cows.

In a recent study, ovariectomized, nonpregnant, and nonlactating cows that were treated with corticotropin to trigger endogenous cortisol release as it occurs around calving were found to respond with an increase in plasma glucose concentration and a concomitant decline in serum [Pi] to a degree similar to what is observed in cows around parturition.[74] This observation suggests that mechanisms independent of milk production, such as hormone-induced redistribution of Pi between intra- and extracellular space or P losses into urine, should be considered factors contributing to periparturient hypophosphatemia. Renal losses of Pi in dairy cattle around parturition are marginal with urine [Pi] ranging considerably below 1 mmol/L.[23,28,67] Assuming a daily urine volume of 20 L, the urine [Pi] would have to increase above 5 mmol/L to explain a decline of the extracellular [Pi] by 0.5 mmol/L.

Occurrence of Hypophosphatemia

Chronic P deficiency can be common in grazing animals in arid regions with low P content in soil. More acute and transient episodes of hypophosphatemia and P depletion are often seen in dairy cows around parturition and in early lactation.

Hypophosphatemia is a common finding in periparturient recumbent cattle but also in sick but ambulatory as well as in clinically healthy periparturient cattle.[75–84] The incidence of hypophosphatemia in periparturient dairy cows is considerable. A large British data set, including serum biochemical results of several thousand clinically healthy dairy cows, found an incidence of hypophosphatemia of more than 15% in cows between 0 to 9 days in milk and of approximately 10% in cows between 10 and 20 days in milk.[81,82] A German data set, including serum biochemical results of blood samples collected on the first day after calving of more than 7000 clinically healthy dairy cows, revealed an incidence of severe hypophosphatemia (serum [Pi] < 0.5 mmol/L or 1.5 mg/dL) of 1.2%, mild to moderate hypophosphatemia (0.5 mmol/L or 1.5 mg/dL < serum [Pi] < 1.6 mmol/L or 4.9 mg/dL) of 52.7%, normophosphatemia (1.6 mmol/L or 4.9 mg/dL < serum [Pi] < 2.3 mmol/L or 7.1 mg/dL) of 39.9%, and hyperphosphatemia (serum [Pi] > 2.3 mmol/L or 7.1 mg/dL) of 6.2%.[83] With a majority of healthy periparturient dairy cows categorized as hypophosphatemic based on this widely accepted reference range, the investigator reasonably questions the validity of this reference range for early periparturient cows.[83]

The reported incidences of hypophosphatemia in recumbent periparturient dairy cows with or without concomitant hypocalcemia range between 66% and

93%.[77,79,83,85] Although it seems that the incidence of hypophosphatemia is higher in recumbent than ambulatory periparturient cows, it is under contentious debate whether hyposphosphatemia in recumbent cows is the cause or a consequence (decreased feed intake or decreased gastrointestinal motility) of the disorder.

Few studies have reported the incidence of hypophosphatemia in sick but ambulatory periparturient cattle. These incidences ranged between 35% and 57% and have been attributed primarily to feed intake depression.[66,83]

Clinical Signs Associated with Hypophosphatemia

A plethora of clinical signs and conditions, such as unthriftiness, anorexia, pica, impaired growth and fertility, muscle weakness and recumbency, intravascular hemolysis, osteomalacia, and many others, have been associated with P deficiency in ruminants. Because signs attributed to chronic P depletion differ from acute P deficiency, it seems reasonable to differentiate between these forms. While bone demineralization, decreased growth, and fertility are primarily associated with chronic P deficiency, muscle weakness, recumbency or intravascular hemolysis has been reported in acutely hypophosphatemic individuals.[13,54,78,86]

Although hypophosphatemia is frequently used as a synonym for P depletion, it can be assumed that most of these signs are considered indicative of total P depletion or depletion of the Pi pool rather than of hypophosphatemia per se. There is little evidence suggesting that hypophosphatemia without concomitant P depletion has any deleterious effects.

Chronic P depletion caused by long-term ingestion of P-deficient diets or ingestion of compounds binding P in the gastrointestinal tract is characterized by anorexia, pica, unthriftiness, poor growth or weight loss, impaired fertility and milk production, and most of all bone demineralization leading to rickets or osteomalacia. The primary effect of P depletion on the organism seems to be anorexia. Other clinical signs often associated with P deficiency, such as weight loss and decreased fertility and productivity, are likely the result of energy and nutrient deficiency ensuing from decreased feed intake.[3,39,54,87–89] Several studies have reported that there is no beneficial effect on fertility or milk production of feeding P in excess of recommended requirements.[39,90]

Acute hypophosphatemia in fresh cows is of particular importance to the dairy industry. Apart from feed intake depression, hypophosphatemia in early lactating cows has been associated with clinical signs and syndromes, such as the downer cow syndrome or periparturient hemoglobinuria.[78,80,86,87] In particular, the empiric observation that hypophosphatemia seems more common or more pronounced in recumbent periparturient cows unresponsive to IV Ca infusion than in cows responding to IV Ca administration has led to the widely held assumption that hypophosphatemia may be a causative or at least contributing factor to the so-called downer cow syndrome.[78–80,84,85] Nonetheless, experimentally decreasing plasma [Pi] to values as low as 0.3 mmol/L (0.9 mg/dL) by limiting dietary P intake did not result in recumbency or signs of muscle weakness or disturbed muscle function and recumbent cows with hypophosphatemia do not consistently respond to oral or parenteral Pi supplementation.[4,91,92] It must be emphasized, however, that models inducing hypophosphatemia by reducing dietary P uptake result in a gradually developing P depletion and, therefore, are poorly suited to mimic the sudden decline of plasma [Pi] at the onset of lactation when a dramatic increase of the P drain through the udder results in a sudden disequilibrium of P homeostasis, potentially overwhelming regulatory mechanisms. It is worthwhile to consider the possibility that clinical signs may not be caused by subnormal serum [Pi] or intracellular P or Pi content per se but rather by the kinetics of the decline of the intracellular P content, not allowing enough time for counter-regulation.

In human medicine, the negative effects of P depletion on muscle function are well established. Severe hypophosphatemia in humans has been associated with muscle pain, muscle weakness, impaired cardiac contractility, and impaired respiratory muscle strength—clinical signs that have effectively been treated with oral or parenteral P supplementation.[54,93–96] The mechanisms through which P depletion impairs muscle function have not yet been identified but several potential mechanisms have been proposed, as follows:

- ATP and creatine phosphate deficiency due to inadequate intracellular Pi content
- Impaired cell membrane stability due to decreased availability of phospholipids
- Hampered glycolysis and glycogenolysis due to inadequate intracellular P required for phosphorylation
- Shift of the hemoglobin-O_2 dissociation curve leading to tissue hypoxia due to a shift of intracellular acid-base equilibrium resulting from intracellular P depletion

In dogs, P depletion was shown to result in a decrease of muscle tissue P content that was associated with a decrease of the transmembrane potential of muscle cells, which is likely to affect the excitability of muscle cells.[56]

Although the unequivocal proof for the causative association between recumbency due to impaired muscle strength and P depletion in cattle is still missing, the evidence discussed previously corroborates this hypothesis.

Intracellular ATP depletion is also the presumed cause of intravascular hemolysis, which is occasionally observed in dairy cows in early lactation, a condition commonly called postparturient hemoglobinuria (PPH).[86] A decrease in intracellular ATP content in erythrocytes can increase osmotic fragility of the erythrocytes and may result in intravascular hemolysis in severe cases.[92] After inducing hypophosphatemia in cows by limiting the dietary P supply, however, self-limiting hemoglobinemia but not hemoglobinuria was observed.[92] The understanding of the etiology of this condition is further obscured by animals suffering from PPH not consistently responding to parenteral supplementation of PO_4 salts.[86,97] Other causes, such as copper deficiency, increased oxidative stress, ketosis, acidosis, and unidentified hemolysing substances contained in plants, such as the sugar beet, have been discussed as alternative or contributing causes. The discrepancy between the high incidence of periparturient hypophosphatemia and the negligible incidence of PPH make it unlikely that P deficiency is anything more than a contributing factor to PPH.

Impaired phagocytic activity of leukocytes has been associated with intracellular ATP depletion in hypophosphatemic states in the human literature.[98,99] Granuloyctes diminished chemotactic and phagocytic function in individuals with severe hypophosphatemia resulting from parenteral carbohydrate administration. These abnormalities resolved when patients were treated with P. The potential effect of P depletion on leukocyte function in cattle has thus far received little attention.[100]

Treatment Indication

Although there is no debate over the need to supplement cattle that have been fed rations with inadequate P content over an extended time period, the rationale for treatment of acute hypophosphatemia is under contentious debate. The main reason for the controversy is not only the lack of unequivocal evidence for the association between hypophosphatemia and some of the signs and symptoms associated with it but also the lack of evidence unambiguously documenting a positive effect of P supplementation in clinical cases. The debate primarily centers around whether and to what extent hypophosphatemia actually reflects P depletion, to what extent hypophosphatemia is of clinical relevance, and whether hypophosphatemia is the cause or rather the consequence or even just an incidental finding in a sick cow.

Treatment of hypophosphatemia occurring concomitantly with periparturient hypocalcemia is not required in most instances because parenteral Ca administration also increases the serum [Pi], presumably through a negative feedback on PTH release and enhanced gastrointestinal motility after treatment of hypocalcemia.[12,68] In sick anorectic patients, P supplementation is considered unnecessary when the primary cause of feed intake depression can be resolved in a timely manner.[66] Based on the research currently available, there is strong evidence to recommend supplementing oral P to chronically P-depleted ruminants; however, only moderate evidence exists to justify the treatment of acute hypophosphatemia. Evidence for the effect of the treatment on the primary symptom or syndrome (eg, recumbency or intravascular hemolysis) is variable but oral P supplementation, when done correctly, presents minimal risk for patients and could, therefore, be considered a treatment option. Parenteral treatment, in contrast, presents certain trade-offs between benefit and harm, which should be taken into account before opting for this treatment approach (discussed later).

Frequently the decisions of if and how acute hypophosphatemia is treated are based on the personal experience and preference of the attending veterinarian. The author is a strong proponent of oral P supplementation as supportive treatment in anorectic patients that do not adequately respond to the treatment of the primary condition causing feed intake depression. Ongoing anorexia may exacerbate feed intake depression, resulting in a vicious circle affecting the P homeostasis and potentially hampering the recovery of the patient.[87–89,91]

Treatment of Hypophosphatemia

For P supplementation in ruminants, either oral or parenteral treatment has been proposed. Although aggressive IV treatment is rarely necessary, a veterinarian may choose this route under certain circumstances (eg, when severe intravascular hemolysis is believed caused by hypophosphatemia).

Parenteral Treatment

Compounds for parenteral phosphate supplementation

The efficacy of IV treatment primarily depends on the P-containing compound used. For metabolism and cell function, the organism requires P as inorganic PO_4. Monosodium dihydrogen PO_4 (NaH_2PO_4) and disodium monohydrogen PO_4 (Na_2HPO_4) are the best-studied PO_4 salts, with well-documented efficacy to correct hypophosphatemia in cattle and other species after IV infusion.[101–106] Potassium PO_4 salts (either monobasic or dibasic) are used for parenteral P supplementation in humans and companion animals in intensive care but require constant monitoring of the serum potassium concentration.[104] Potassium PO_4 salt solutions cannot be administered as bolus, as is commonly done with sodium PO_4 salts under field conditions, because this could result in potentially life-threatening hyperkalemia. Currently in Europe and the United States, there are no pharmaceutical products containing PO_4 salts approved for IV treatment in food animal species, making the use of PO_4 salts an extralabel treatment.

PO_4 salts have limited solubility at neutral pH and tend to precipitate when mixed with other minerals, such as Ca or Mg.[105] To circumvent this solubility problem, the pharmaceutical industry often uses more soluble P-containing compounds for parenteral treatment of hypophosphatemia. Such compounds are, for example, phosphite (PO_2), hypophosphite (PO_3), and organic substances, such as sodium glycerophosphate, butafosfan (butylamino-methylethyl-phosphoric acid), toldimfos (dimethylamino-methylphenyl-phosphinate or 4-dimethylamino-2-methylphenyl phosphinic acid), and aminoethyl dihydrogen PO_4. To be metabolically utile, these compounds have to be converted into PO_4 after administration and before being cleared from the organism. Of the compounds listed, only sodium glycerophosphate is rapidly hydrolyzed into glycerol and PO_4, thereby resulting in a rapid increase in serum [Pi].[102,106,107] For the other substances, a pathway of conversion into PO_4 has not been identified. Studies exploring the pharmacokinetics of toldimfos and buta-fosfan and their effect on the serum [Pi] failed to document an immediate or protracted effect on the serum [Pi]. Although a certain time delay could be anticipated because of the required hydrolyzation of the molecule to release PO_4, the clearance rates for these substances suggest that conversion to PO_4 does not occur in quantitatively relevant amounts. For toldimfos, more than 95% of the unchanged substance could be recovered from different excretions of treated animals within 48 hours of treatment.[108] For butafosfan, more than 75% of the unchanged substance was found excreted in urine within 12 hours of treatment.[109] Rapid renal excretion has also been reported for PO_3 that failed to alter the serum [Pi] in the 12 hours after treatment in cattle.[101,102,105] The author is not aware of any studies documenting the efficacy of aminoethyl dihydrogen PO_4 to correct hypophosphatemia in cattle.

Dosage recommendations

With Pi a predominantly intracellular electrolyte and the serum [Pi] a poor surrogate parameter to estimate the extent of P depletion, it is practically impossible to determine the precise amount of Pi required to restore the P balance by IV treatment. Different empirically based dosage recommendations for cattle ranging from 13 to 20 mg P/kg body weight (ie, 0.4–0.7 mmol/kg) have been proposed.[68,106,110] These doses recommended for cattle are slightly above doses used in hypophosphatemic humans.[103,111] Doses used in cattle and other species are difficult to compare because the entire dose is typically administered as a bolus for reasons of practicality, whereas Pi infusions in other species are administered as a drip to prevent hyperphosphatemia and phosphaturia.

The dose range proposed previously corresponds to between 7 and 12 g of Pi administered IV to an adult cow. In the literature, a preparation of either 300 mL aqua bidest (distilled water), containing 30 g anhydrous NaH_2PO_4, or 500 mL aqua bidest (distilled water), containing the equivalent of 36 g of anhydrous Na_2HPO_4, has been proposed as a single dose for an adult cow (both equivalent to approximately 8 g of P).[68,106,110,112] The subcutaneous administration of such custom-made solutions has also been proposed in the past but this route of administration should be strongly discouraged because unbuffered NaH_2PO_4 or Na_2HPO_4 solutions at the concentration, suggested previously, have a pH below 3.5 and above 9.5, respectively, and thus are likely to cause tissue irritation.[110]

Pharmaceutical products with butafosfan as P source contain the equivalent of 17.4 mg P/mL in a P form that does not seem metabolically utile. A label dose does not even provide 0.5 g of P for a 600-kg cow, which cannot measurably increase the serum [Pi].[113] Similarly, the recommended dose of products containing toldimfos (2–8 mg/kg) or aminoethyl dihydrogen PO_4 (1.5 g per treatment) contains less than 0.6 g P per dose for a 600-kg cow.

When using sodium glycerophosphate, the equivalent of 56 g of the anhydrous form of this compound is required to provide the equivalent to 8 g of P to a 600-kg cow. Infusion solutions containing sodium glycerophosphate in combination with Ca-gluconate are commercially available but contain sodium glycerophosphate in the range of 10 to 20 g per single dose.[102,106] This dose may suitable to support the P balance but is inadequate to correct severe hypophosphatemia that is the only indication for parenteral treatment.

Infusion rate

The administration of sodium PO_4 salt solutions, described previously, has been recommended and is often done as IV bolus infusion.[13,106,110,112] Although the author is not aware of any published report of clinical complications that may have occurred during or after PO_4 salt infusion in cattle, the rapid infusion presents the main concern of IV correction of hypophosphatemia with PO_4 salts. Bolus infusion of either NaH_2PO_4 or Na_2HPO_4 to cattle at the proposed dose led on average to increases of the serum [Pi] by more than 3 mmol/L (9.3 mg/dL), resulting in peak concentrations of more than 4.5 mmol/L (14 mg/dL).[101,102] Although short-lived, this transient hyperphosphatemia may have several implications of potentially clinical relevance: because of the limited solubility of P, this mineral tends to precipitate as either Ca-PO_4 or Mg-PO_4 once the [Pi] in extracellular fluid increases above the physiologic range. The ensuing (although mild to moderate) decline of the serum Ca concentration that is well documented in cattle presents a potential risk for any subclinically hypocalcemic cow.[102,105] Soft tissue mineralization has also been discussed as a possible side effect of hyperphosphatemia but is likely only an issue if repeated doses are administered.[114]

Administering PO_4 salts as bolus infusion furthermore results in serum [Pi] above the renal threshold for Pi that was reported at approximately 2.3 mmol/L (7 mg/dL) in cattle.[115] Peak [Pi] far above this renal threshold results in substantial renal Pi excretion, which shortens the plasma half-life of the administered P and translates to a treatment effect that would only last between 2 and 4 hours.[101,102,105,115] Lowering the infusion rate by extending the infusion period to 1 to several hours would address all of these issues.

Because of the short treatment effect, it is evident that parenteral P supplementation cannot under any circumstances be a stand-alone treatment approach but rather needs to be combined with oral P supplementation. Veterinarians have to balance the benefit of raising the serum [Pi] within minutes but for a short time against the possible harm resulting from a decline in serum Ca concentration [Ca] to determine whether IV bolus infusion is justified and indicated.

Recommendations for parenteral treatment

Currently the best established recommendation for IV treatment in cattle is the administration of either 30 g of anhydrous NaH_2PO_4 dissolved in 300 mL of sterile deionized water or 36 g of anhydrous Na_2HPO_4 (or 90 g of $Na_2HPO_4 \times 12\ H_2O$) dissolved in 500 mL of sterile deionized water and administered as slow IV infusion. Because products approved for the use in cattle are frequently not available, this treatment would have to be administered in an extralabel manner.

Treatment with sodium glycerophosphate is effective in correcting hypophosphatemia but products approved for parenteral use in cattle containing this compound are infusion solutions designed to treat hypocalcemia. They do not provide enough PO_4 per treatment dose to correct marked hypophosphatemia.

Other organic compounds used and recommended for the treatment of hypophosphatemia, such as butafosfan, toldimfos, and aminoethyl dihydrogen PO_4, must be considered unsuitable for this purpose because the label dose does not provide nearly enough P and the compounds seem rapidly cleared from the body rather than being converted into PO_4.

Oral Treatment

Oral Pi supplementation in cattle was shown an effective treatment approach to correct hypophosphatemia and P depletion.[101,116–118] For the treatment of acute hypophosphatemia where rapid absorption of PO_4 is essential, the solubility characteristics of the specific PO_4 salt are important. NaH_2PO_4 is the most commonly used compound for this purpose, with well-documented efficacy to restore serum [Pi].[101,116–118] Treatment failures have been reported, with Na_2HPO_4 providing equivalent amounts of P.[119] Although differences between both salts could be due to the lower solubility of Na_2HPO_4, the study reporting a lack of efficacy was conducted on animals that were not P deficient and on a normal diet, which is likely to have confounded the results.[119]

Dicalcium phosphate is commonly used to effectively supplement chronically P-deficient animals where a sustained but not necessarily rapid treatment effect is required. The poor solubility characteristics of this compound nonetheless result in a protracted treatment effect after oral administration as a drench or bolus, making this salt unsuitable for rapid correction of P deficiency.[101,118] Monocalcium phosphate is more soluble than dicalcium phosphate, and oral administration of 240 g of monocalcium phosphate monohydrate was effective in increasing the serum [Pi] for up to 12 hours, although the effect was less pronounced than after treatment with NaH_2PO_4, providing the same amount of Pi (Grünberg, 2014). Potassium salts, in particular monopotassium phosphate, are used in humans and companion animals to treat hypophosphatemia that is frequently associated with hypokalemia in anorectic patients. This salt may also be suitable to treat hypophosphatemic and hypokaleimic cattle orally, but the author is not aware of any study having determined treatment effect and appropriate doses for monopotassium phosphate in cattle.

Dosage recommendations for sodium PO_4 in cattle range from 150 to 230 g of NaH_2PO_4 or 180 to 270 g of anhydrous N_2HPO_4 administered orally, which is equivalent to between 40 and 60 g of Pi. These dosage recommendations are empiric but seem adequate to restore serum [Pi] in mildly to moderately hypophosphatemic cows for at least 8 to 12 hours.[101,118] The adequacy of this dose for severely hypophosphatemic animals does not seem to have been confirmed.

Studies investigating the kinetics of Pi absorption from the gastrointestinal tract after oral administration of NaH_2PO_4 yield inconsistent results. Although some investigators report a time to peak concentration of serum [Pi] after oral treatment of 3 to 4 hours, in 1 study, peak serum [Pi] was within 1 hour of treatment.[101,116–118] Because absorption of P from the forestomachs does not seem to occur in biologically relevant amounts, rumen motility is assumed an important factor affecting treatment efficacy.[118]

A potential concern associated with oral treatment using PO_4 salts, particularly when administered repeatedly, is the possible interference of high [Pi] in rumen fluid with the absorption rate of other minerals, such as Ca or Mg from the rumen. Due to the limited solubility of Pi, precipitation of Pi as quanite ($MgNH_4PO_4.6H_2O$) or calcium phosphate may occur with excessive concentrations.[120] Precipitation of Mg in the reticulorum decreases the bioavailability of this mineral and can, therefore, present a risk for animals with marginal or inadequate dietary Mg supply. In small ruminants, Mg absorption from the reticulorumen was found to decrease with ruminal [Pi] above 38 mmol/L. A study conducted in pregnant heifers found that a ration containing excessive amounts of P (0.64%) decreased intestinal P absorption.[121] In dairy cattle treated with 300 g NaH_2PO_4 orally, rumen [Pi] at or above this threshold was measured for at least 2 hours after treatment. Rumen [Ca] in that study was found decreased for at least 4 hours post-treatment.[118]

In summary, oral NaH_2PO_4 seems to provide the most appropriate treatment to rapidly correct P depletion and hypophosphatemia in dairy cows, Doses of 150 to 230 g per adult cow are effective to increase the serum [Pi] concentration within 3 to 4 hours of treatment and last for at least 8 to 12 hours. Treatment could, therefore, be repeated in 12- to 24-hour intervals when indicated. In patients with severe hypophosphatemia or rumen atony, monitoring the treatment effect on the serum [Pi] is warranted. Although treatment with 200 to 400 g of monocalcium phosphate might be a suitable alternative in mildly to moderately hypophosphatemic animals, dicalcium phosphate is not suitable to rapidly correct hypophosphatemia in cattle.

HYPERPHOSPHATEMIA
Phosphorus Toxicity and Hyperphosphatemia

With ruminant diets limited in their P content and P-containing supplements expensive, P toxicity is uncommon in ruminants. Supplying ruminants with excessive amounts of P orally results in decreased intestinal P absorption and, thereby, increased fecal P excretion. Excessive dietary P levels in growing animals fed a high-concentrate diet result in increased salivary and renal Pi excretion in the first place. Depending on the urine pH that determines the solubility of urine Pi, hyperphosphaturia may result in the formation of urinary calculi. Alkaline urine in ruminants on a diet rich in P predisposes to formation of struvite (ammonium magnesium phosphate) and apatite (calcium phosphate) crystals. Acidic urine may increase renal P excretion through a mechanism, termed *titratable acidity*, but the low urine pH improves solubility, thereby reducing the risk of formation of PO_4 crystals.[49,50]

In transition cows, overfeeding P can have deleterious effects by disturbing the regulation of the Ca homeostasis. With high dietary P supply, the body downregulates the intestinal P absorption by inhibiting the hydroxylation of vitamin D_3 to its active form. Because vitamin D_3 regulates not only intestinal P but also the Ca absorption, the ability of the periparturient cow on a high-P diet to respond to disturbances of the Ca homeostasis around calving is impaired.[122] Dry cow rations with a dietary P content above 0.5% increase the risk of clinical hypocalcemia presumably through the mechanism described previously.[123] High dietary P was also reported to have a negative affect on intestinal Mg absorption, which further predisposes to periparturient hypocalcemia.[121,124]

Acute hyperphosphatemia in ruminants is seen most commonly as a consequence of dehydration and ensuing hemoconcentration. Dehydration can cause hyperphosphatemia not only by reducing the plasma volume but also by decreasing saliva and urine production and in lactating cows by decreasing milk production. Although ruminants in contrast to monogastric species do not depend on proper renal function for Pi excretion, with dehydration, the serum [Pi] may exceed the renal threshold, in which case decreased renal perfusion can exacerbate hyperphosphatemia.[125,126] Furthermore, severe dehydration is often associated with decreased peripheral tissue perfusion and ensuing lactic acidosis. As discussed previously, acidemia impairs the cellular P uptake, thereby potentially contributing to the development of hyperphosphatemia.[26,127]

Hyperphosphatemia is a common finding in cattle with right displaced abomasum or abomasal volvulus and was found associated with the degree of dehydration.[66] Presumably because dehydration in these cases is associated with feed intake depression and rumen stasis, serum [Pi] in affected animals rarely exceeds 3.0 mmol/L (9.3 g/dL). Hyperphosphatemia in dehydrated cattle is not considered a primary problem requiring therapeutic intervention but rather a symptom of dehydration.

Hyperphosphatemia can occur as a consequence of massive releases of intracellular P after rhabdomyolysis or hemolysis. Muscle damage not only results in leakage of intracellular P but also other predominantly intracellular compounds, such as potassium, myoglobin, or enzymes like aspartate aminotransferase, creatine kinase, and lactate dehydrogenase that all have elevated serum concentration or activity. A concomitant decline in serum [Ca] that is frequently observed in patients with rhabdomyolysis and has been attributed to the deposition of Ca as Calcium phosphate salts in damaged muscle tissue.[128] In patients with rhabdomyolysis, hyperphosphatemia can be exacerbated by disturbed renal function that is a common complication of myoglobinuria.

Marked hyperphosphatemia in ruminants has been reported after parenteral administration of sodium PO_4 salt solutions given as IV bolus or after overdose of PO_4 enemas.[101,102,105,129] Peak serum [Pi] reported after IV bolus infusion of doses recommended for cattle were above 4 mmol/L (13 mg/dL) but were short-lived and not associated with any clinically apparent complications. Mild to moderate declines in serum [Ca] (in the range of 0.1–0.5 mmol/L or 0.5–2 mg/dL) and mild declines of the serum Mg concentration [Mg] (less than 0.1 mmol/L or 0.25 mg/dL) lasting for 2 to 4 hours were observed.[102,105]

Adverse effects of sodium PO_4–based laxatives as either oral or enema preparations have been reported in humans and companion animals as well as in 1 case in a pigmy goat.[129–131] Sodium PO_4 is shown rapidly and effectively absorbed through the mucosa of the colon in humans and animals. In cattle, intra-abomasal infusion of a standard oral dose of sodium PO_4, thus bypassing the rumen (230 g NaH_2PO_4), resulted in a peak serum [Pi] of more than 3.2 mmol/L (9.9 mg/dL) within 1 hour that was accompanied by a decline of the serum [Ca] by 0.3 mmol/L (1.2 mg/dL).[118] These observations underscore not only the effectiveness of enteral Pi absorption, particularly when bypassing the rumen, but also the risk of adverse effects when inadvertently or accidentally overdosing sodium PO_4 salts.

Severe hyperphosphatemia from sodium PO_4 administration is associated with hypocalcemia, hypernatremia, hypokalemia, hyperglycemia, severe metabolic acidosis (when using NaH_2PO_4), and hyperosmolality.[130–132]

Clinical Signs of Hyperphosphatemia

In most cases, clinical and subclinical signs observed with hyperphosphatemia are not due to the supranormal concentrations of this electrolyte in serum or the body P pool per se but rather to the interference of hyperphosphatemia with the regulation of other electrolytes, namely Ca and possibly Mg. Chronic P oversupply has clinically relevant effects on Ca metabolism through inhibition of renal vitamin D_3 hydroxylation that reduces intestinal Ca absorption and Ca deposition primarily as Calcium phosphate crystals in soft tissue.[133] Secondary hyperparathyroidism with excessive bone resorption occurs and urolithiasis and soft tissue mineralization may develop.

Particularly in the late stages of pregnancy, excessive dietary P supply increases the risk for clinical periparturient hypocalcemia.[122] High dietary P content has also been associated with reduced intestinal Mg absorption, which may further contribute to the risk of clinical hypocalcemia because Mg increases PTH receptor affinity.[121]

Acute hyperphosphatemia resulting from parenteral administration of phosphate salts does not seem to cause clinical signs as long as the serum [Pi] does not exceed 7.5 mmol/L (23 mg/dL) in humans.[130,131] Accidental IV administration of PO_4 salt solutions to children resulted in peak serum [Pi] in the range of 4.5 mmol/L (14 mg/dL) without obvious clinical complications.[134] P concentrations above 7.5 mmol/L

(23 mg/dL) were accompanied by severe clinical signs, including depressed consciousness or coma, seizures, and spontaneous tetanic contractions, in humans and animals.[131,135–137] Hypocalcemia is likely the major cause for muscle fasciculation and tetanic contractions.[137] The most dramatic clinical signs, those of neurologic dysfunction, are probably not directly associated with high P concentration but rather caused by the considerable increase in plasma osmolality resulting from high plasma Na and P concentrations.[132]

Treatment of Hyperphosphatemia

In cases of chronic dietary oversupply of P, reducing the dietary P content is the first and most effective treatment approach. Because adjustment of the metabolism to the modified diet may take time, supplying additional Ca to compensate for the negative effects on the Ca homeostasis has been recommended. Supplementing dietary Ca also reduces the risk of urolithiasis in sheep on a high-P diet.[138] For treatment of urolithiasis causing urinary tract obstruction, readers are referred to publications addressing this subject specifically.[139] Prevention and control measures for urolithiasis consist of reducing the dietary P supply as much as possible while supplementing dietary Ca with the objective to obtain a Ca to P ratio of 1.2:1 to 2:1.[140] Supplementation of the diet with acidogenic salts, such as ammonium chloride or ammonium sulfate, lowers the urinary pH, thereby increasing the solubility of urine Pi.[139] Other measures include stimulation water intake (addition of salts to the diet) to dilute urine and stimulation of salivation, by increasing the dietary roughage content, to facilitate Pi excretion through saliva.

Treatment of severe and acute hyperphosphatemia is indicated only when clinical signs are apparent and should target at the alleviation of clinical signs. Hypocalcemia is considered the most important complication and should be corrected by parenteral administration of Ca-gluconate solutions. Ca should only be substituted to control clinical symptoms, not to completely correct hypocalcemia because extra Ca stimulates soft tissue mineralization.[137] Parenteral administration of isotonic fluids help reduce serum osmolality and serum [Pi] and Na concentration. Correction of acid-base equilibrium is indicated with severe acidemia. The use of hypertonic solutions, particularly when based on Na, must be avoided because these exacerbate plasma hypertonicity and worsen hypernatremia. The use of 5% dextrose solutions has been proposed to trigger a shift of Pi into the intracellular space.[137] Because affected patients often are hyperglycemic and acidosis blunts the serum [Pi]–lowering effect of insulin, this treatment may not be of much use.

REFERENCES

1. Hill SR, Knowlton KF, Kebreab E, et al. A model of phosphorus digestion and metabolism in the lactating dairy cow. J Dairy Sci 2008;91:2021–32.
2. Karn JF. Phosphorus nutrition of grazing cattle: a review. Anim Feed Sci Tech 2001;89:133–53.
3. NRC. Minerals. In: National Academies Press, editor. Nutrient requirements of dairy cattle. 7th edition. Washington, DC: National Acadamy of Science; 2001. p. 109–17.
4. Breves G, Schroder B. Comparative aspects of gastrointestinal phosphorus metabolism. Nutr Res Rev 1991;4:125–40.
5. Bryant MP, Robinson IM, Chu H. Observations on the nutrition of bacteroides-succinogenes – A ruminal cellulolytic bacterium. J Dairy Sci 1959;42:1831–47.

6. Burroughs W, Latona A, Depaul P, et al. Mineral influences upon urea utilization and cellulose digestion by rumen microorganisms using the artificial rumen technique. J Anim Sci 1951;10:693–705.
7. Bevington A, Mundy KI, Yates AJ, et al. A study of intracellular ortho-phosphate concentrationin human muscle and erythrocytes by P-31 nuclear magnetic resonance spectroscopy and selective chemical assay. Clin Sci 1986;71:729–35.
8. Butterworth PJ. Phosphate homeostasis. Mol Aspects Med 1987;9:289–386.
9. Grummer RR, Davis CL. Plasma-concentration and lipid-composition of lipopro-teins in lactating dairy cows fed control and high grain diets. J Dairy Sci 1984; 67:2894–901.
10. Sevinc M, Basoglu A, Guzelbektas H, et al. Lipid and lipoprotein levels in dairy cows with fatty liver. Turk J Vet Anim Sci 2003;27:295–9.
11. Contreras GA, O'Boyle NJ, Herdt TH, et al. Lipomobilization in periparturient dairy cows influences the composition of plasma nonesterified fatty acids and leukocyte phospholipid fatty acids. J Dairy Sci 2010;93:2508–16.
12. Grünberg W. Phosphorus homeostasis in dairy cattle. Some answers, more questions: Dairy Nutrition Conference. Fort Wayne, April 22–23, 2008, p. 29–35.
13. Goff JP. Pathophysiology of calcium and phosphorus disorders. Vet Clin N Am Food Anml Pract 2000;16:319–38.
14. Maekawa M, Beauchemin KA, Christensen DA. Chewing activity, saliva produc-tion, and ruminal pH of primiparous and multiparous lactating dairy cows. J Dairy Sci 2002;85:1176–82.
15. Cassida KA, Stokes MR. Eating and resting salivation in early lactating dairy cows. J Dairy Sci 1986;69:1282–92.
16. Castillo AR, St-Pierre NR, del Rio NS, et al. Mineral concentrations in diets, wa-ter, and milk and their value in estimating on-farm excretion of manure minerals in lactating dairy cows. J Dairy Sci 2013;96:3388–98.
17. Cerbulis J, Farrell HM. Composition of milks of dairy cattle. 2. Ash, calcium, magbnesium, and phosphorus. J Dairy Sci 1976;59:589–93.
18. Klop G, Ellis JL, Bannink A, et al. Meta-analysis of factors that affect the utiliza-tion efficiency of phosphorus in lactating dairy cows. J Dairy Sci 2013;96: 3936–49.
19. Morse D, Head HH, Wilcox CJ, et al. Effects of concentration of dietary phos-phorus on amount and route of excretion. J Dairy Sci 1992;75:3039–49.
20. Neville MC, Peaker M. Secretion of calcium and phosphorus into milk. J Physiol 1979;290:59–67.
21. House WA, Bell AW. Mineral accretion in the fetus and adnexia during late gestation in Holstein cows. J Dairy Sci 1993;76:2999–3010.
22. Horst RL. Regulation of calcium and phosphorus homeostasis in the dairy cow. J Dairy Sci 1986;69:604–16.
23. Grünberg W, Donkin SS, Constable PD. Periparturient effects of feeding a low dietary cation-anion difference diet on acid-base, calcium, and phosphorus ho-meostasis and on intravenous glucose tolerance test in high-producing dairy cows. J Dairy Sci 2011;94:727–45.
24. Werner A, Kinne RK. Evolution of the Na-P-i cotransport systems. Am J Physiol Regul Integr Comp Physiol 2001;280:R301–12.
25. Virkki LV, Biber J, Murer H, et al. Phosphate transporters: a tale of two solute car-rier families. Am J Physiol Renal Physiol 2007;293:F643–54.
26. Mackler B, Lichtenstein H, Guest GM. Effects of ammonium chloride acidosis on glucose tolerance in dogs. Am J Physiol 1952;168:126–30.

27. Grünberg W, Morin DE, Drackley JK, et al. Effect of continuous intravenous administration of a 50% dextrose solution on phosphorus homeostasis in dairy cows. J Am Vet Med Assoc 2006;229:413–20.
28. Grünberg W, Morin DE, Drackley JK, et al. Effect of rapid intravenous administration of 50% dextrose solution on phosphorus homeostasis in postparturient dairy cows. J Vet Intern Med 2006;20:1471–8.
29. Body JJ, Cryer PE, Offord KP, et al. Epinephrine is a hypophosphatemic hormone in man. Physiological effects of circulating epinephrine on plasma calcium, magnesium, phosphorus, parathyroid hormone and calcitonin. J Clin Invest 1983;71:572–8.
30. Gold LW, Massry SG, Arieff AI, et al. Renal bicarbonate wasting during phosphate depletion – Possible cause of altered acid-base homeostasis in hyperparathyroidism. J Clin Invest 1973;52:2556–62.
31. Wright RD, Blairwest JR, Nelson JF, et al. Handling of phosphate by a parotid gland (ovine). Am J Physiol 1984;246:F916–26.
32. Schroder B, Kappner H, Failing K, et al. Mechanisms of intestinal phosphate transport in small ruminants. Br J Nutr 1995;74:635–48.
33. Shirazi-Beechey SP, Penny JI, Dyer J, et al. Epithelial phosphate transport in ruminants, mechanisms and regulation. Kidney Int 1996;49:992–6.
34. Lee DB, Walling MW, Brautbar N. Intestinal phosphate absorption – Influence of vitamin D and non-vitamin D factors. Am J Physiol 1986;250:G369–73.
35. Escoubet B, Djabali K, Amiel C. Adaptation to Pi deprivation of cell Na-dependent Pi uptake. A widespread process. Am J Physiol 1989;256:C322–8.
36. Blum JW, Fischer JA, Hunziker WH, et al. Parathroid hormone responses to catecholamines and to changes of extracellular calcium in cows. J Clin Invest 1978; 61:1113–22.
37. Hirsch PF, Baruch H. Is calcitonin an important physiological substance? Endocrine 2003;21:201–8.
38. Berndt TJ, Schiavi S, Kumar R. "Phosphatonins" and the regulation of phosphorus homeostasis. Am J Physiol Renal Physiol 2005;289:F1170–82.
39. Call JW, Butcher JE, Shupe JL, et al. Clinical effects of low dietary phosphorus concentrations in feed given to lactating dairy cows. Am J Vet Res 1987;48: 133–6.
40. Williams SN, McDowell LR, Warnick AC, et al. Phosphorus concentration in blood, milk, feces, bone, and selected fluids and tissues of growing heifers as affected by dietary phosphorus. Livest Res Rur Develop 1991. Available at: http://www.lrrd.org/lrrd3/2/florida4.htm. Accessed September 1, 2013.
41. Rodehutscord M, Pauen A, Windhausen P, et al. Effects of drastic changes in P-intake on P concentration in blood and rumen fluid of lactating ruminants. J Vet Med A 1994;41:611–9.
42. Sharifi K, Mohri M, Rakhshani A. The relationship between blood indicators of phosphorus status in cattle. Vet Clin Pathol 2007;36:354–7.
43. Meinkoth JH, Allison RW. Sample collection and handling: getting accurate results. Vet Clin North Am Small Anim Pract 2007;37:203–19.
44. Breves G, Rosenhagen C, Holler H. Saliva secretion of inorganic phosphorus in phosphorus-depleted sheep. J Vet Med A 1987;34:42–7.
45. Valk H, Sebek LB, Beynen AC. Influence of phosphorus intake on excretion and blood plasma and saliva concentrations of phosphorus in dairy cows. J Dairy Sci 2002;85:2642–9.
46. Scott D, McLean AF, Buchan W. The effect of variation in phosphorus intake on net intestinal phosphorus absorption, salivary phosphorus secretion and

pathway of excretion in sheep fed roughage diets. Q J Exp Physiol Cogn Med Sci 1984;69:439–52.

47. Puggaard L, Kristensen NB, Sehested J. Effect of decreasing dietary phosphorus supply on net recycling of inorganic phosphate in lactating dairy cows. J Dairy Sci 2011;94:1420–9.

48. Osbaldiston GW, Moore WE. Renal function tests in cattle. J Am Vet Med Assoc 1971;159:292–301.

49. Tolgyesi G. Renal phosphorus excretion of cattle and its relationship with calcium supply. Acta Vet Acad Sci Hung 1972;22:25–9.

50. Lunn DP, McGuirk SM. Renal regulation of electrolyte and acid-base balance in ruminants. Vet Cln N Am Food Anim Pract 1990;6:1–28.

51. Read MV, Engels EA, Smith WA. Phosphorus and the grazing ruminant. 4. Blood and fecal grab samples as indicators of the P-status of cattle. S Afr J Anim Sci 1986;16:18–22.

52. de Waal HO, Koekemoer GJ. Blood, rib bone and rumen fluid as indicators of phosphorus status of grazing beef cows supplemented with different levels of phosphorus at Armoedsvlakte. S Afr J Anim Sci 1997;27:76–84.

53. Little DA. Definition of an objective criterion of body phosphorus reserves in cattle and its evaluation in vivo. Can J Anim Sci 1984;64:229–31.

54. Knochel JP. Hypophosphatemia. Clin Nephrol 1977;7:131–7.

55. Kemp GJ. Abnormalities of P(I) concentration in plasma and cells. Clin Chem 1993;39:2028–31.

56. Fuller TJ, Carter NW, Barcenas C, et al. Reversible changes of muscle cell in experimental phosphorus deficiency. J Clin Invest 1976;57:1019–24.

57. Hettleman BD, Sabina RL, Drezner MK, et al. Defective adenosine-triphosphate synthesis – An explanation for skeletal muscle dysfunction in phosphate deficient mice. J Clin Invest 1983;72:582–9.

58. Pough DG. Normal values and conversions. In: Pugh DG, editor. Sheep and goat medicine. 1st edition. Philadelphia: WB Saunders; 2002. p. 451–3.

59. Roussel JD, Aranas TJ, Seybt SH. Metabolic profile testing in Holstein cattle in Louisiana – Reference values. Am J Vet Res 1982;43:1658–60.

60. Tumbleson M, Wingfield W, Johnson HD, et al. Serum electrolyte concentration as a function of age, in female dairy cattle – Aging and serum electrolytes. Cornell Vet 1973;63:58–64.

61. Teleni E, Dean H, Murray RM. Some factors affecting measurement of blood inorganic phosphorus in cattle. Aust Vet J 1976;52:529–33.

62. Parker BN, Blowey RW. Comparison of blood from jugular vein and coccygeal artery and vein of cows. Vet Rec 1974;95:14–8.

63. Gelfert CC, Staufenbiel R. Proper sampling and handling of blood samples to secure reliable results for the diagnosis of metabolic disturbances in cattle. Prakt Tierarzt 1998;79:640–50.

64. Montiel L, Tremblay A, Girard V, et al. Preanalytical factors affecting blood inorganic phosphate concentration in dairy cows. Vet Clin Pathol 2007;36:278–80.

65. Palmer LS, Cunningham WS, Eckles CH. Normal variation in the inorganic phosphorus of the blood of dairy cattle. J Dairy Sci 1930;13:174–95.

66. Grünberg W, Constable P, Schroder U, et al. Phosphorus homeostasis in dairy cows with abomasal displacement or abomasal volvulus. J Vet Intern Med 2005;19:894–8.

67. Husband J, Burnell M, Plate P, et al. Metabolic disturbances associated with left displaced abomasum (LDA) in the first month post calving: a case-controlled study. Cattle Practice 2013;21:62–5.

68. Goff JP. Treatment of calcium, phosphorus, and magnesium balance disorders. Vet Clin North Am Food Anim Pract 1999;15:619–39.
69. Adrogue HJ, Chap Z, Okuda Y, et al. Acidosis-induced glucose intolerance is not prevented by adrenergic blockade. Am J Physiol 1988;255:E812–23.
70. Mak RH. Effect of metabolic acidosis on insulin action and secretion in uremia. Kidney Int 1998;54:603–7.
71. Bigner DR, Goff JP, Faust MA, et al. Acidosis effects on insulin response during glucose tolerance tests in Jersey cows. J Dairy Sci 1996;79:2182–8.
72. Robertson A, Marr A, Moodie EW. Milk fever. Vet Rec 1956;68:173–80.
73. Goff JP, Kimura K, Horst RL. Effect of mastectomy on milk fever, energy, and vitamins A, E, and beta-carotene status at parturition. J Dairy Sci 2002;85: 1427–36.
74. Kim D, Yamagishi N, Devkota B, et al. Effects of cortisol secreted via a 12-h infusion of adrenocorticotropic hormone on mineral homeostasis and bone metabolism in ovariectomized cows. Domest Anim Endocrinol 2012;43:264–9.
75. Rohn M, Tenhagen BA, Hofmann W. Survival of dairy cows after surgery to correct abomasal displacement: 1. Clinical and laboratory parameters and overall survival. J Vet Med A 2004;51:294–9.
76. Kalaitzakis E, Panousis N, Roubies N, et al. Macromineral status of dairy cows with concurrent left abomasal displacement and fatty liver. N Z Vet J 2010;58: 307–11.
77. Metzner M, Klee W. Clinical signs and blood parameters in recumbent dairy cows with special reference to serum phosphate levels. Tierarztl Umsch 2005; 60:13–22.
78. Menard L, Thompson A. Milk fever and alert downer cows: does hypophosphatemia affect the treatment response? Can Vet J 2007;48:487–91.
79. Stolla R, Schulz H, Martin R. Changes in the clinical picture of parturient paresis. Tierarztl Umsch 2000;55:295–9.
80. Gerloff BJ, Swenson EP. Acute recumbency and marginal phosphorus deficiency in dairy cattle. J Am Vet Med Assoc 1996;208:716–9.
81. Macrae AI, Whitaker DA, Burrough E, et al. Use of metabolic profiles for the assessment of dietary adequacy in UK dairy herds. Vet Rec 2006;159:655–61.
82. Macrae AI, Burrough E, Forrest J. Assessment of nutrition in dairy herds: use of metabolic profiles. Cattle Practice 2012;20:120–7.
83. Staufenbiel R. Neue Aspekte zum klinischen Bild und zur Therapie der Gebaerparese des Rindes. Vet Med Rev 2002;26:12 V6.
84. Hofmann W, el-Amrousi S. Studies on bovine paresis. 5. Experiments on the medicamentous therapy of hypophosphoremia and paresis in atypical parturient paresis. Dtsch Tierarztl Wochenschr 1971;78:156–9 [in German].
85. Bostedt H, Wendt V, Prinzen R. Peripartal paresis of the milk clinical and biochemical aspects. Prakt Tierarzt 1979;60:18–34.
86. Jubb TF, Jerrett IV, Browning JW, et al. Hemoglobinuria and hypophosphatemia in postparturient dairy cows without dietary deficiency of phosphorus. Aust Vet J 1990;67:86–9.
87. Milton JT, Ternouth JH. Phosphorus metabolism in ruminants. 2. Effects of inorganic phosphorus concentration upon food intake and digestibility. Aust J Agr Res 1985;36:647–54.
88. Ternouth JH, Sevilla CC. The effects of low levels of dietary phosphorus upon the dry matter intake and metabolism of lambs. Aust J Agr Res 1990;41:175–84.
89. Gartner RJ, Murphy GM, Hoey WA. Effects of induced subclinical phosphorus deficiency on feed intake and growth of beef heifers. J Agric Sci 1982;98:23–9.

90. Wu Z, Satter LD. Milk production and reproductive performance of dairy cows fed two concentrations of phosphorus for two years. J Dairy Sci 2000;83: 1052–63.
91. Valk H, Sebek LB. Influence of long-term feeding of limited amounts of phosphorus on dry matter intake, milk production, and body weight of dairy cows. J Dairy Sci 1999;82:2157–63.
92. Ogawa E, Kobayashi K, Yoshiura N, et al. Hemolytic anemia and red blood cell metabolic disorders attributable to low phosphorus intake in cows. Am J Vet Res 1989;50:388–92.
93. Lotz M, Zisman E, Bartter FC. Evidence for a phosphorus depletion syndrome in man. N Engl J Med 1968;278:409–15.
94. Davis SV, Olichwier KK, Chakko SC. Reversible depression of myocardial performance in hypophosphatemia. Am J Med Sci 1988;295:183–7.
95. Hasselstrom L, Wimberley PD, Nielsen VG. Hypophosphatemia and acute respiratory failure in a diabetic patient. Intensive Care Med 1986;12:429–31.
96. Newman JH, Neff TA, Ziporin P. Acute respiratory failure associated with hypophosphatemia. N Engl J Med 1977;296:1101–3.
97. Mullins JC, Ramsay WR. Haemoglobinuria and anaemia associated with aphosphorosis. Aust Vet J 1959;35:140–7.
98. Craddock PR, Yawata Y, Vansante L, et al. Acquired phagocyte dysfunction resulting from parenteral hyperalimentation. N Engl J Med 1974;290:1403–7.
99. Kiersztejn M, Chervu I, Smogorzewski M, et al. On the mechanisms of impaired phagocytosis in phosphate depletion. J Am Soc Nephrol 1992;2:1484–9.
100. Mullarky IK, Wark WA, Dickenson M, et al. Short communication: analysis of immune function in lactating dairy cows fed diets varying in phosphorus content. J Dairy Sci 2009;92:365–8.
101. Cheng YH, Goff JP, Horst RL. Restoring normal blood phosphorus concentrations in hypophosphatemic cattle with sodium phosphate. Vet Med 1998;93: 383–8.
102. Horner S, Staufenbiel R. The influence of different therapeutic substances applieable for phosphat substitution on the concentration of phosphore in the blood. Prakt Tierarzt 2004;85:666–73.
103. Charron T, Bernard F, Skrobik Y, et al. Intravenous phosphate in the intensive care unit: more aggressive repletion regimens for moderate and severe hypophosphatemia. Intensive Care Med 2003;29:1273–8.
104. Willard MD, DiBartola SP. Disorders of phosphorus. In: DiBartola SP, editor. Fluid therapy in small animal practice. 2nd edition. Philadelphia: WB Saunders; 2000. p. 163–74.
105. Sachs M, Hurwitz S. The efficacy of calcium and hypophosphite in raising plasma calcium and inorganic phosphate levels in the blood of normal dairy cows. Refu Vet 1972;29:153–8.
106. Staufenbiel R, Dallmeyer M, Horner S. Hinweise zur Therapie des atypischen Festlegens. Proc. 2. Leipziger Tierärztekongress. Leipzig, Germany, January 17–9, 2002. p. 288–91.
107. Topp H, Hochfeld O, Bark S, et al. Glycerophosphate Is Interchangeable with Inorganic phosphate in terms of safety and serum pharmacokinetics. Pharmacology 2011;88:193–200.
108. EMEA. Committee for veterinary medicinal products. Toldimfos. Summary report. EMEA/MRL/717/99-Final. 1999. Available at: http://www.ema.europa.eu/docs/en_GB/document_library/Maximum_Residue_Limits_-_Report/2009/11/WC500015617.pdf. Accessed September 1, 2013.

109. EMEA. Committee for veterinary medicinal products. Butafosfan (Extension to lactating cows). Summary report (2). EMEA/MRL/734/00-Final. April 2000. Available at: http://www.ema.europa.eu/docs/en_GB/document_library/Maximum_Residue_Limits_-_Report/2009/11/WC500011128.pdf. Accessed September 1, 2013.

110. McGaughan CJ. Treatment of mineral disorders in cattle. Vet Clin North Am Food Anim Pract 1992;8:107–45.

111. Perreault MM, Ostrop NJ, Tierney MG. Efficacy and safety of intravenous phosphate, replacement in critically ill patients. Ann Pharmacother 1997;31:683–8.

112. Constable P. Fluid and electrolyte therapy in ruminants. Vet Clin North Am Food Anim Pract 2003;19:557–97.

113. Rollin E, Berghaus RD, Rapnicki P, et al. The effect of injectable butaphosphan and cyanocobalamin on postpartum serum beta-hydroxybutyrate, calcium, and phosphorus concentrations in dairy cattle. J Dairy Sci 2010;93:978–87.

114. Alfrey AC, Ibels LS. Role of phosphate and pyrophosphate in soft tissue calcification. Adv Exp Med Biol 1978;103:187–93.

115. Symonds HW, Manston R. Response of bovine kidney to increasing plasma inorganic phosphorus concentrations. Res Vet Sci 1974;16:131–3.

116. Braun U, Dumelin J, Liesegang A, et al. Effect of intravenous calcium and oral sodium phosphate on electrolytes in cows with parturient paresis. Vet Rec 2007;161:490–2.

117. Braun U, Bryce B, Liesegang A, et al. Efficacy of oral calcium and/or sodium phosphate in the prevention of parturient paresis in cows. Schweiz Arch Tierheilkd 2008;150:331–8.

118. Grünberg W, Dobbelaar P, Breves G. Kinetics of phosphate absorption in lactating dairy cows after enteral administration of sodium phosphate or calcium phosphate salts. Br J Nutr 2013;110:1012–23.

119. Horner S, Staufenbiel R. About the effictiveness of orally or subcutaneous phosphorus substitution with cattle. Prakt Tierarzt 2004;85:761–7.

120. Dua K, Care AD. Impaired absorption of magnesium in the etiology of grass tetany. Br Vet J 1995;151:413–26.

121. Schonewille JT, Vantklooster AT, Beynen AC. High phosphorus intake depresses apparent magnesium absorption in pregnant heifers. J Anim Physiol Anim Nutr 1994;71:15–21.

122. Reinhardt TA, Conrad HR. Mode of action of pharmacological doses of cholecalciferol during parturient hypocalcemia in dairy cows. J Nutr 1980;110:1589–96.

123. Jorgensen NA. Combating milk fever. J Dairy Sci 1974;57:933–44.

124. Goff JP. Macromineral disorders of the transition cow. Vet Clin North Am Food Anim Pract 2004;20:471–94.

125. Watts C, Campbell JR. Biochemical changes following bilateral nephrectomy in the bovine. Res Vet Sci 1970;11:508–14.

126. Watts C, Campbell JR. Further studies on effects of total nephrectomy in bovine. Res Vet Sci 1971;12:234–45.

127. Oster JR, Alpert HC, Vaamonde CA. Pathogenesis of Hyperphosphatemia in Lactic-Acidosis - Disparate Effects of Racemic (Dl-)Lactic and Levo (L-)Lactic Acid on Plasma Phosphorus Concentration. Can J Physiol Pharmacol 1985; 63:1599–602.

128. Akmal M, Goldstein DA, Telfer N, et al. Resolution of muscle calcification in rhabdmomyolysis and acute renal failure. Ann Intern Med 1978;89:928–36.

129. Hickman SA, Gill MS, Marks SL, et al. Phosphate enema toxicosis in a pygmy goat wether. Can Vet J 2004;45:849–51.

130. Jorgensen LS, Center SA, Randolph JF, et al. Electrolyte abnormalities induced by hypertonic phosphate enemas in 2 cats. J Am Vet Med Assoc 1985;187: 1367–8.

131. Marraffa JM, Hui A, Stork CM. Severe hyperphosphatemia and hypocalcemia following the rectal administration of a phosphate-containing Fleet (R) pediatric enema. Pediatr Emerg Care 2004;20:453–6.

132. Atkins CE, Tyler R, Greenlee P. Clinical, biochemical, acid-base, and electrolyte abnormalities in cats after hypertonic sodium phosphate enema administration. Am J Vet Res 1985;46:980–8.

133. Tanaka Y, Deluca HF. Control of 25-hydroxyvitamin-D metabolism by inorganic phosphorus. Arch Biochem Biophys 1973;154:566–74.

134. Biarent D, Brumagne C, Steppe M, et al. Acute phosphate intoxication in 7 infants under parenteral nutrition. JPEN J Parenter Enteral Nutr 1992;16:558–60.

135. Craig JC, Hodson EM, Martin HC. Phosphate enema poisoning in children. Med J Aust 1994;160:347–51.

136. Martin RR, Lisehora GR, Braxton M, et al. Fatal poisoning from sodium phosphate enema – Case report and experimental study. J Am Med Assoc 1987; 257:2190–2.

137. Helikson MA, Parham WA, Tobias JD. Hypocalcemia and hyperphosphatemia after phosphate enema use in a child. J Pediatr Surg 1997;32:1244–6.

138. Bushman DH, Emerick RJ, Embry LB. Experimentally induced ovine phosphatic urolithiasis – relationships involving dietary calcium phosphorus and magnesium. J Nutr 1965;87:499–504.

139. Larson BL. Identifying, treating, and preventing bovine urolithiasis. Vet Med 1996;91:366–77.

140. Udall RH, Chow FH. The etiology and control of urolithiasis. Adv Vet Sci Comp Med 1969;13:29–57.

Fluid Therapy in Calves

Geof W. Smith, DVM, MS, PhD[a],*, Joachim Berchtold, Dr Med Vet[b]

KEYWORDS

- Fluid therapy • Calves • Diarrhea • Strong ion acidosis

KEY POINTS

- Early and aggressive fluid therapy is critical in correcting the metabolic complications associated with calf diarrhea in order to avoid deaths.
- Oral electrolyte therapy can be used with success in calves, but careful consideration should be given to the type of oral electrolyte used.
- Electrolyte solutions with high osmolalities (>650 mOsm/L) have been shown to significantly slow abomasal emptying and can be a risk factor for abomasal bloat in calves.
- Milk should not be withheld from calves with diarrhea for more than 12 to 24 hours.
- Hypertonic saline and hypertonic sodium bicarbonate can be used effectively for intravenous fluid therapy on farms when intravenous catheterization is not possible.
- A simplified fluid therapy protocol using only 5-L bags of saline and 8.4% hypertonic sodium bicarbonate provides optimal resuscitation for both beef and dairy calves with diarrhea, dehydration, and moderate to severe acidosis.

Neonatal diarrhea remains the most common cause of death in both beef and dairy calves. Despite significant progress in understanding the pathophysiology of neonatal diarrhea, it continues to be a major cause of economic loss to the cattle industry. A complete review of the pathophysiology of diarrhea is beyond the scope of this article and has recently been covered elsewhere in the literature.[1] Some pathogens cause secretory diarrhea, causing the small intestine to move from a net absorption of fluid to a net secretion of chloride, sodium, and water into the intestinal lumen. This increase in secretion overwhelms the absorptive capacity of the large intestine, resulting in diarrhea. Other pathogens damage the small intestinal villi, which results in failure to absorb electrolytes and water (malabsorptive diarrhea). However, regardless of the pathogen or the mechanism involved, diarrhea increases the loss of electrolytes and water in the feces of calves and often decreases milk intake. This process results in dehydration, strong ion acidosis, electrolyte abnormalities (usually decreased sodium and increased or decreased potassium), increased D-lactate concentrations,

The authors have nothing to disclose.
[a] Population Health and Pathobiology, North Carolina State University, Raleigh, 1060 William Moore Drive, Raleigh, NC 27607, USA; [b] Tierärztliche Praxis, Dr. Berchtold, Strassberg 6, Pittenhart 83132, Germany
* Corresponding author.
E-mail address: geoffrey_smith@ncsu.edu

and a negative energy balance (from anorexia and malabsorption of nutrients). Therefore diarrhea is by far the most common indication for fluid therapy in neonatal calves. The primary goals of treating calf diarrhea are as follows:

1. Correct free water and electrolyte abnormalities
2. Correct acid-base deficits (acidemia)
3. Provide nutritional support
4. Eliminate and/or prevent *Escherichia coli* bacteremia.

Three of these 4 goals can be met with fluid therapy. This article provides an overview of fluid therapy in calves with particular emphasis on treating diarrhea. Practical options for fluid therapy that can be performed on the farm are emphasized.

ORAL ELECTROLYTE THERAPY

According to the World Health Organization (WHO), the development of oral rehydration therapy was one of the most significant advances in human medicine of twentieth century. Oral electrolyte solutions also continue to serve as the backbone of treatment protocols for diarrhea in neonatal calves because they are cheap and easy to administer on farms. Oral electrolyte solutions are indicated in any diarrheic calf that has at least a partially functional gastrointestinal tract. If oral electrolyte solutions are administered to a calf with ileus, the fluid pools in the forestomach, resulting in bloat and rumen acidosis. In general, a calf with any sort of suckle reflex or that shows any chewing action can be considered to safely tolerate oral fluids.

Oral electrolyte therapy in calves was thoroughly reviewed in a previous issue of *Veterinary Clinics of North America: Food Animal Practice*[2]; however, a brief overview is warranted here. Oral electrolyte solutions were originally developed in human medicine for treatment of diarrhea associated with cholera infection, with the original WHO electrolyte formulation based on the following main principles[3]:

1. It was an isotonic solution that contained an approximately equimolar mixture of sodium (90 mM/L) and glucose (2%).
2. It contained potassium because of the severe potassium depletion associated with diarrhea and anorexia.
3. It contained glycine to facilitate absorption of sodium, glucose, and water.
4. It contained bicarbonate to correct the metabolic acidosis associated with diarrhea.

Although much research has been done on oral fluid therapy since that time, little progress has been made from the original principles of the 1960s.

Considerable variability exists in the quality of commercial oral electrolyte solutions that are currently available (**Table 1**) and practitioners must put some thought into the product they choose to use in practice. As was eloquently stated in a previous article by Michell and colleagues,[4] simply recommending oral electrolyte rehydration in this decade is as imprecise as advocating antibiotics would be without considering the drug or condition being treated. There are several important factors to consider when deciding on a product. Current knowledge indicates that an oral electrolyte solution must satisfy the following 4 requirements: (1) supply sufficient sodium to normalize the extracellular fluid (ECF) volume; (2) provide agents (glucose, citrate, acetate, propionate, or glycine) that facilitate absorption of sodium and water from the intestine; (3) provide an alkalinizing agent (acetate, propionate, or bicarbonate) to correct the acidosis usually present in calves with diarrhea; and (4) provide energy, because most calves with diarrhea are in a state of negative energy balance.[2] A brief discussion of factors to consider when choosing an oral electrolyte solution is warranted.

Table 1
A comparison of oral electrolyte products available in North America

	Sodium (mM/L)	Potassium (mM/L)	Chloride (mM/L)	Strong Ion Difference	Alkalinizing Agent	Total Osmolality (mOsm/L)
Advance Arrest (Milk Specialties, Fond du Lac, WI, USA)[a]	46	7	30	23	Bicarbonate (12 mM/L)	245
Bounce Back (Manna Pro, Chesterfield, MO, USA)[a]	136	10	112	34	Bicarbonate (48 mM/L)	—
Blue Ribbon Calf Electrolytes (Merrick, Middleton, WI, USA)[a]	144	20	75	89	None	390
Bovine Bluelite C (Techmix, Stewart, MN, USA)	59	24	56	27	None	269
Calf-Lyte II (Vetoquinol, Lure, France)	112	15	43	84	Acetate (80 mM/L)	428
Calf-Lyte II HE (Vetoquinol, Lure, France)	112	15	43	84	Acetate (80 mM/L)	726
Calf Quencher (Vedco, St Joseph, MO, USA)	142	24	80	86	Bicarbonate (86 mM/L)	731
Deliver (AgriLabs, St Joseph, MO, USA)[a]	67	16	49	34	Bicarbonate (36 mM/L)	305
Diaque (Boehringer Ingelheim, Fort Dodge, IA, USA)	90	15	55	50	Bicarbonate (25 mM/L) and acetate (12 mM/L)	377
Electrolyte-F-Calf (Bio Agri Mix, Mitchell, ON, Canada)	92	15	43	64	Acetate (60 mM/L)	385
Entrolyte HE (Zoetis, Florham Park, NJ, USA)	106	26	51	81	Bicarbonate (80 mM/L)	739
Epic calf electrolyte (Bioniche, Belleville, ON, Canada)	92	30	45	77	Acetate (52 mM/L)	360
Hydrafeed (A&L Laboratories, Minneapolis, MN, USA)	110	10	40	80	Bicarbonate (80 mM/L)	380
Hydralyte (Vet-A-Mix and AgriLabs, St Joseph, MO, USA)	90	30	45	75	Acetate (60 mM/L)	614
Land O Lakes Base plus Add Pack (Land O Lakes, St Paul, MN, USA)	119	23	56	86	Acetate (51 mM/L and citrate (10 mM/L)	455
Land O Lakes Complete (Land O Lakes, St Paul, MN, USA)	121	20	78	64	Bicarbonate (38 mM/L)	490
Resorb (Zoetis, Florham Park, NJ, USA)	75	25	80	20	None	315
Revibe HE (Zoetis, Florham Park, NJ, USA)	120	20	50	90	Acetate (80 mM/L)	466
Revitilyte (Vets Plus Inc, Menomonie, WI, USA)	110	50	20	140	Bicarbonate (90 mM/L)	577
VitaLyte Plus (Vita Plus Corp, Madison, WI, USA)	150	31	45	136	Bicarbonate (80 mM/L)	527

This listing does not include every product available in North America. No discrimination or specific endorsement of any product is intended.
[a] Signifies that data were calculated from product label instead of provided by the manufacturer. In some cases there was insufficient information on the label to provide an exact calculation so values may be inexact.

Sodium Concentration

Sodium is the osmotic skeleton of the ECF and therefore of plasma. Because sodium is the principal determinant of the volume of the ECF, it must be present in an oral electrolyte solution to rapidly correct the losses that have occurred with dehydration and diarrhea. The ideal sodium concentration for oral rehydration therapy in calves is not completely known, but most research suggests it should be between 90 and 130 mM/L. Products containing sodium at lower concentrations are not able to adequately correct dehydration. Oral electrolyte products with very high sodium concentrations might be expected to cause hypernatremia and have also been shown to delay abomasal emptying rates because of increased osmolality.[5]

Chloride Concentration

Although calves lose chloride during diarrhea, this loss does not occur to the same degree as for sodium.[6] A general guideline has been that oral electrolyte products should contain chloride in concentrations between 40 and 80 mEq/L.

Potassium Concentration

Like sodium and chloride, potassium is lost in the feces of calves with diarrhea. Therefore all calves with diarrhea have a total body deficit of potassium.[7] However, in acute cases of diarrhea calves may have increased blood potassium concentrations (hyperkalemia). With dehydration, aldosterone is released from the pituitary gland. Aldosterone acts on the kidney to conserve sodium and water at the expense of increased potassium losses. Therefore, in chronic cases of diarrhea, calves can have profound depletion of body potassium stores and generally have low serum concentrations of potassium. Clinical signs of hypokalemia include profound muscular weakness, which is often present in calves with chronic diarrhea. General recommendations are that oral electrolyte products used in calves with diarrhea contain potassium concentrations between 10 and 30 mM/L.

Sodium Absorption

Sodium absorption by the small intestine is a passive process, and is linked to the movement of actively absorbed or secreted solutes. If sodium is present in the lumen of the small intestine without either glucose or amino acid, there is either a small net absorption or no net sodium movement across the jejunum.[8] One of the earliest mechanisms of intestinal sodium absorption to be discovered was linked with sugar.[9] Glucose can be cotransported with sodium from the intestinal lumen to the inside of the enterocyte at the brush border membrane.[8] Because this mechanism was well understood by the 1960s, almost all early oral electrolyte formulations were mixtures of sodium and glucose. Neutral amino acids such as glycine, alanine, or glutamine can also facilitate sodium absorption in the small intestine by a mechanism similar to that of glucose. Whether amino acids are needed in addition to glucose in oral electrolyte solutions is not well understood, but the addition of glycine seems to further improve water absorption in the intestine. In addition, volatile fatty acids such as acetate or propionate have been shown to facilitate sodium absorption in the gut.[10,11] The mechanism by which volatile fatty acids stimulate sodium absorption in the intestine seems to be different from that of glucose or amino acids. Therefore acetate seems to have an additive effect to glucose and amino acids, meaning that a significant increase in intestinal sodium absorption can be expected in electrolyte products containing volatile fatty acids, even when they already contain high concentrations of glucose and/or glycine.

Osmolality

Commercially available oral electrolyte products in North America can range from roughly isotonic (280–300 mOsm/L) to extremely hypertonic (700–800 mOsm/L). The primary difference in most of these products is the amount of glucose that is added. Because of a countercurrent exchange mechanism in the small intestine, the effective osmolality at the tip of the intestinal villus is about 600 mOsm/L.[12] Therefore, clinicians can take advantage of solutions that have higher energy levels. In contrast, low-osmolality fluids (<350 mOsm/L) generally have lower energy content because they have limited glucose. High-osmolality solutions provide greater nutritional support to calves relative to lower osmolality products and have not been shown to cause detrimental effects, particularly in relation to maintaining hydration status, intestinal osmolality, serum glucose concentrations, and intestinal flow rate.[13] Research has shown that milk replacer is better able to maintain normal serum glucose concentration than either hypertonic or isotonic oral electrolyte solutions.[14] However, as expected, oral electrolyte solutions rehydrated calves and prevented the development of metabolic acidosis more effectively than did milk replacer because they have a higher sodium concentration. Multiple studies have shown that high-osmolality oral electrolyte solutions maintain higher serum glucose and lower β-OH butyrate (ketone) concentrations than lower osmolality electrolyte solutions.[14,15] Research has also shown that when calves were deprived of milk, those fed low-osmolality oral electrolyte solutions had significantly greater weight loss than calves fed high-osmolality oral electrolytes.[16]

With the principle that hypertonic oral electrolytes supply more energy to calves than isotonic osmolality products, the next question becomes what osmolality that might cause deleterious effects? Although the research available to date does not provide a good answer to that question, there are indications that electrolyte solutions with extremely high osmolalities (>700–750 mOsm/L) and glucose concentrations might cause problems. A product with an osmolality greater than what is already present in the intestinal lumen could worsen diarrhea. Most calves with enteric pathogens already have hypersecretion of electrolytes and water into the small intestinal lumen, which could be exacerbated with the feeding of extremely hypertonic solutions (electrolyte or milk replacer). Increasing the intraluminal tonicity would increase the secretion of water and electrolytes into the intestinal lumen, thus increasing the severity of diarrhea. This effect would likely be magnified with severe villus damage, which is often present in diarrheic calves.

Oral electrolyte solutions with extremely high osmolalities have also been shown to slow abomasal emptying rates compared with isotonic products.[5,17,18] Calves fed an oral electrolyte solution with a total osmolality of 360 mOsm/L had a significantly faster abomasal emptying rate than calves fed a solution with an osmolality of 717 mOsm/L.[18] This finding suggests that electrolyte products with very high osmolality (or high glucose concentrations) would be likely to induce abomasal ileus, thus increasing the risk of bloat and/or abomasitis. Abomasal bloat is a syndrome in young calves that is characterized by anorexia, abdominal distension, bloat, and often death in 6 to 48 hours. This condition occurs most commonly in dairy calves and seems to have a sporadic occurrence with some farms having multiple outbreaks at times. The abomasal bloat syndrome was experimentally reproduced by drenching young Holstein calves with a carbohydrate mixture containing milk replacer, corn starch, and glucose mixed in water.[19] The investigators proposed that the pathophysiology of abomasal bloat is primarily excess fermentation of high-energy gastrointestinal contents. Gas-producing bacteria such as *Clostridium perfringens*, *Sarcina ventriculi*, or *Lactobacillus* species have also been thought to play a role in this syndrome.[19,20]

Although the exact pathogenesis of abomasal bloat is not completely understood, the disease is likely to be mutifactorial in origin.[21] Having large amounts of fermentable carbohydrate present in the abomasum (from milk, milk replacer, or high-energy oral electrolyte solutions) along with the presence of fermentative enzymes (produced by bacteria) is likely to lead to gas production and bloat. This process would be exacerbated by anything that slowed abomasal emptying or caused gastrointestinal ileus. Feeding extremely high-osmolality electrolyte products and/or milk replacers has been noted to be a risk factor on some farms for the development of abomasal bloat in calves (data not published), so although the ideal osmolality of an oral electrolyte solution for calves is not completely understood, a moderate-osmolality solution (400–600 mOsm/L) would be ideal in dairy calves or in beef calves that have been separated from the dam. If milk is to be withheld for any length of time, a hypertonic oral electrolyte solution should be indicated to provide energy to the calf. However, lower osmolality solutions might be appropriate for beef calves that are still suckling or in conjunction with milk replacer in dairy calves that maintain a good appetite. The authors recommend avoiding extremely high-osmolality oral electrolyte products (>700 mOsm/L) for the reasons stated earlier.

Alkalinizing Ability

Acidemia and metabolic acidosis occur in almost all cases of calf diarrhea. These conditions were originally attributed to bicarbonate loss in the feces along with a decreased glomerular filtration rate in response to severe dehydration.[22,23] However, more recent data in calves with diarrhea have indicated that the acidosis in calves with diarrhea results from differences in strong ion balance.[6] This is discussed in more detail in article by Lorenz and colleagues and the article by Constable elsewhere in this issue. Research into intravenous (IV) fluid therapy protocols has indicated that severely acidemic calves are unable to correct their metabolic acidosis when rehydrated with nonalkalinizing solutions.[24] Therefore it is imperative that either oral or IV fluid therapy protocols be able to increase blood pH. This has classically been done by adding alkalinizing agents (ie, bicarbonate, acetate, or propionate) to oral electrolyte mixtures. More recently, there has been growing interest in studying the strong ion difference (SID) of electrolytes as they relate to the efficacy of a different product to promote alkalinization. In practice, both (having an alkalinizing agent and a high SID) are likely important.

Acetate, propionate, bicarbonate, and citrate are all considered alkalinizing agents and are frequently present in commercial oral electrolyte solutions. Bicarbonate-containing fluids are effective at correcting a severe acidosis, because bicarbonate reacts directly with H^+ ions to form CO_2 and H_2O. Acetate and propionate are also alkalinizing agents and have been shown to have alkalinizing effects similar to bicarbonate.[25–27] Acetate and propionate are only effective alkalinizing agents when they are metabolized; a process that forms water and creates bicarbonate ions (bicarbonate precursors). This metabolic process seems to still function efficiently in calves with severe diarrhea because the alkalinizing ability of the acetate has been shown to be as effective as bicarbonate.[26] Acetate and propionate have several advantages compared with bicarbonate:

a. As discussed earlier, acetate and propionate facilitate sodium and water absorption in the calf small intestine, whereas bicarbonate does not.
b. Acetate and propionate produce energy when metabolized, whereas bicarbonate does not.
c. Acetate and propionate do not alkalinize the abomasum, whereas bicarbonate does; low abomasal pH is a natural defense mechanism against bacterial proliferation.

Gastric acidity is a well-accepted barrier to colonization and infection of the gastro-intestinal tract by bacteria, and is a primary defense mechanism against pathogens that are ingested orally.[28] Bacteria such as *E coli* and *Salmonella* are killed at a gastric pH between 2.5 and 3.0, whereas they multiply at a pH greater than 5.0.[29,30] Therefore maintaining a low abomasal pH is critical to avoid colonization of the intestinal tract with pathogenic bacteria in calves. The feeding of oral electrolyte products containing bicarbonate has been shown to alkalinize the abomasum in calves.[25–27] Suckling of bicarbonate-containing oral electrolyte solutions can cause a large and sustained in-crease in abomasal pH (**Fig. 1**). A similar effect is not seen with acetate-based products.[25,27] Abomasal acidity provides a natural barrier to ingested bacteria, and maintaining a low abomasal pH decreases the number of viable coliform bacteria that reach the small intestine. This process increases nonspecific resistance to intestinal colonization. Therefore the increase in abomasal pH seen with electrolyte products that contain high concentrations of bicarbonate may facilitate growth of bacterial diarrheal pathogens and thus increase the severity, duration, and mortality associated with diarrhea in calves.

Strong ion theory is a different approach to acid-base abnormalities and is covered in detail in article by Constable elsewhere in this issue. Based on strong ion theory, it is not necessarily imperative that an electrolyte solution contain an alkalinizing agent to correct metabolic acidosis, but the product must deliver an excess of strong cations (Na^+) relative to the concentration of strong anions (Cl^-). Therefore it has been advo-cated to consider the SID of an oral electrolyte solution when choosing a product. This SID can be calculated as follows: $[Na^+] + [K^+] - [Cl^-] = SID$. Although there has not

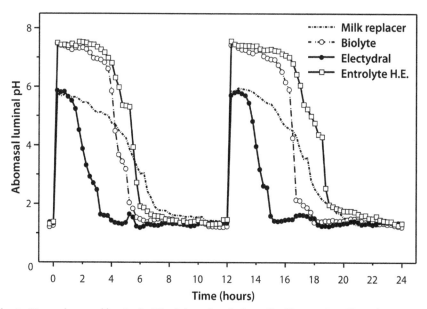

Fig. 1. Mean abomasal luminal pH in dairy calves fed an all-milk protein milk replacer or 1 of 3 oral electrolyte solutions: Biolyte, which contains 86 mM/L bicarbonate; Entrolyte HE (Zoe-tis), which contains 80 mM/L bicarbonate; or Electydral (contains 43 mM acetate and 10 mM propionate). Milk or oral electrolyte solutions were fed for a 24-hour period in random or-der at 0 and 12 hours. (*Modified from* Smith GW, Ahmed AF, Constable PD. Effect of orally administered electrolyte solution formulation on abomasal luminal pH and emptying rate in dairy calves. J Am Vet Med Assoc 2012;241:1075–82.)

been any definitive research to determine the optimal or minimum SID that an oral electrolyte product should contain, a minimum SID of 60 to 80 mEq/L is recommended in a calf with diarrhea.

There are therefore 2 different ways of thinking about alkalinizing ability when considering oral electrolyte products in calves. Is it more important to choose a product with an alkalinizing agent (acetate, bicarbonate), or one with a high SID (high sodium concentration relative to chloride)? There is no good answer to this question; to achieve optimal results, both factors are important. Studies with IV fluid therapy have shown that the metabolic acidosis in calves does not resolve just by rehydrating the animal.[24] Several studies in diarrheic calves have shown that oral electrolytes without alkalinizing agents do not correct metabolic acidosis, and can have a mild acidifying effect.[4,31–33] Recovery rates are always higher and mortality always lower in studies that compare an oral electrolyte solution with an alkalinizing agent to with one without.[32,33] Therefore it has generally been accepted that oral electrolyte products should contain 50 to 80 mM/L of an alkalinizing agent.[2]

It is possible to correct metabolic acidosis in a calf without an alkalinizing agent by choosing a product with a high SID. Studies comparing different oral electrolyte solutions that do not contain any alkalinizing agent consistently show that products with higher SIDs have greater alkalinizing effects than products with lower SIDs.[4,34,35] However, to achieve maximum alkalinizing ability from an oral electrolyte product, the author thinks that both elements are important. For example, one study showed there was no difference in the alkalinizing ability of an electrolyte solution that contained 80 mM/L of acetate and had an SID of 90 compared with a product that contained 80 mM/L of bicarbonate and had an SID of 88.[32] However, both products were far superior to an oral electrolyte solution that contained no alkalinizing agent and had an SID of 15. The ideal electrolyte solution for use in calves with diarrhea should contain at least 50 mM/L of an alkalinizing agent (preferably acetate and/or propionate), and have an SID of at least 60 to 80. However, products without alkalinizing agents and with very low SIDs are commonly available in North America and are not ideal for calves with diarrhea.

ADMINISTRATION OF ORAL ELECTROLYTE SOLUTIONS

In general, oral electrolytes should be fed as an extra meal to calves with diarrhea. For example, if calves are normally being fed twice a day (morning and evening), then oral electrolytes can be fed in the middle of the day. If the additional labor required for the extra feeding is not available, then electrolytes can be fed along with milk (particularly those products that contain acetate or very low concentrations of bicarbonate). Some farms prefer to offer diarrheic calves constant access to low-osmolality electrolytes throughout the day. Regardless of the feeding schedule for electrolytes, it is best to continue milk and/or milk replacer in these calves.

Some experts have recommended a rest-the-gut approach to treating calf diarrhea, suggesting that continued milk feeding will worsen the diarrhea. This concept is based on the principle that milk supplies nutrients in the intestines that the bacteria can use as an energy source, which would lead to further maldigestion of nutrients and increased excretion of fluids (thus more diarrhea). Other arguments for withholding milk in calves with diarrhea include a faster healing of the intestines, less opportunity for overgrowth of the intestines with harmful bacteria, and impaired digestion and utilization of milk and/or milk replacer. Despite these ideas, research has shown that milk feeding does not prolong or worsen diarrhea, or speed healing of the intestines. In a study by Garthwaite and colleagues,[36] 42 calves with naturally occurring diarrhea were divided into 3 groups. In 1 group milk was withheld and calves were fed only oral electrolytes, followed by a gradual return to milk after 2 days. In the second group there was partial removal of milk and calves were fed only a small amount (2.5% of body weight for 2 days followed by 5% of body weight for 2 days), along with oral electrolytes. In the third group calves were continued on their full allotment of milk (10% of body weight per day) along with electrolytes. There was no difference in the severity or duration of diarrhea between any of the groups during the study. However, the calves with diarrhea that were fed both milk and oral electrolytes gained more weight than did calves from which milk was withheld for 1 to 2 days. The calves that continued to receive milk gained weight during the study period, whereas calves in the other two groups lost weight. Weight loss in calves limited to only oral electrolyte solutions has been reported in other studies as well.[16,37]

Another study used an experimentally induced model of diarrhea in calves fed either milk (2 L every 12 hours), an isotonic oral electrolyte solution (85 mM glucose), or a hypertonic oral electrolyte solution (330 mM glucose) over a 48-hour period. Serum glucose concentrations were unchanged over the 48-hour period in the calves fed milk, but steadily declined throughout the study in both groups fed only oral electrolytes.[14] Calves fed only electrolytes developed significant increases in β-OH butyrate and nonesterified fatty acid concentrations over the 48-hour period, indicating that these calves were in a profound negative energy balance. A more recent study on a large dairy in Colorado enrolled 360 calves with naturally occurring diarrhea.[37] One group of calves received the oral electrolyte solution Resorb according to label directions (2 feedings of Resorb only twice a day for 2 days and then 1 L of milk mixed with 1 L of Resorb to day 4 or until diarrhea resolved), whereas the other group received Diaque according to the label (1 packet mixed with 2 L of milk twice daily for 2 days and continued if diarrhea persists). The calves in the Diaque group in which milk feeding was continued gained more weight during the diarrhea period, had higher weaning weights, and had a faster resolution of diarrhea. These studies indicate that even hypertonic oral electrolyte products with very high glucose concentrations do not provide sufficient energy to meet the maintenance and growth requirements of a calf. Therefore the recommendation to temporarily discontinue milk feeding in calves with diarrhea is inappropriate. Calves should be maintained on their full-milk diet plus oral electrolytes when possible. If calves are depressed and refuse to suckle, milk can be withheld for 1 feeding (12 hours) and a hypertonic oral electrolyte product substituted. However, milk feeding should always be resumed within 12 hours.

SUMMARY

Oral electrolytes continue to be the hallmark of routine therapy for treating neonatal calf diarrhea. It is important that practitioners are able to assess dehydration accurately and understand how and when to use oral electrolyte products. There are important differences in the formulation of commercially available electrolyte products found both in North America and around the world. All products are not equal and choosing which of these products to use in practice is an important decision. Practitioners should focus on selecting oral electrolyte solutions that satisfy the following 4 requirements: (1) supply sufficient sodium to normalize the ECF volume, (2) provide agents that facilitate absorption of sodium and water from the intestine, (3) correct the acidosis usually present in calves with diarrhea, and (4) provide energy. In addition, an oral electrolyte should not cause any deleterious effects (such as abomasal bloat or abomasal alkalinization). Because veterinarians are often not directly involved with the administration of oral electrolytes to calves, it is important that they examine the electrolyte product being used in their clients' herds and make recommendations when appropriate.

IV FLUID THERAPY

Although oral electrolyte therapy is generally easier to perform on the farm, there are times when the use of IV fluids is critical when trying to resuscitate calves with diarrhea. Like oral electrolytes, IV fluids are given primarily to correct dehydration, electrolyte imbalances, and acidosis, and to reduce the increased D-lactate concentrations often seen with diarrhea. More detailed information about the pathophysiology of dehydration and electrolyte abnormalities can be found in a previous edition of this article[38] and a detailed explanation of strong ion acidosis and increased D-lactate concentrations can be found in the articles by Lorenz and colleagues and Constable elsewhere in this issue.

Assessing the Need for IV Fluid Therapy

The key for ruminant practitioners is to be able to decide whether IV fluid therapy is necessary in sick calves based on clinical examination rather than on laboratory values. Important clinical parameters to guide decision making on fluid therapy are obtained from the evaluation of hydration status and central nervous system (CNS) function. Degree of enophthalmus is the best predictor of dehydration in calves, followed by skin elasticity determined on the neck and thorax.[39] Detailed information on the clinical assessment of hydration status in calves was previously presented.[2] In clinically sick calves, it is important to evaluate hydration status along with other clinical signs. These signs include the ability of the calf to suckle, severity of CNS depression, and whether or not the calf can stand (degree of weakness). These factors in combination are used to determine whether or not IV fluid therapy is indicated.

Blood gas and acid-base status are ideally determined with a portable blood gas analyzer such as the I-Stat System (Abbott Point of Care Inc, Princeton, NJ). However, these laboratory analyzers are expensive and are therefore not used in most practices. Assessment and diagnosis of acidosis from clinical signs is common in bovine practice. The predictive accuracy of the degree of acidosis from clinical signs has varied between studies. The clinical signs of neurologic depression (weakness; ataxia; and decreased menace, suckle, and panniculus reflex) were highly correlated with the severity of metabolic acidosis in calves without dehydration.[40,41] Also in diarrheic calves, signs of CNS depression, ability to stand, and suckling force all correlated well with metabolic acidosis.[41,42] The degree of enophthalmos and peripheral skin temperature are important and obvious signs that determine whether or not IV fluid therapy is indicated; however, they do not correlate with the degree of acidosis.[39–44]

An important discovery was that metabolic acidosis in diarrheic calves varies during the first weeks of life. Naylor[41,42] discovered that metabolic acidosis is less severe during the first week of life than in diarrheic calves older than 8 days. The base deficit in diarrheic calves older than 1 week was almost twice as high as in calves presented with diarrhea during the first week of life. Subsequent studies confirmed that calves with diarrhea more than 1 week of age usually have a higher base deficit.[44–46] From his findings, depression scoring charts were developed for predicting the severity of metabolic acidosis based on body position, strength of suckle reflex, and age of the calf, with corresponding values for base deficit and bicarbonate requirements for the treatment of metabolic acidosis in diarrheic calves less than or more than 8 days of age. These protocols became a popular approach to guide diagnosis and treatment of acidosis in calves with diarrhea, and are presented in common veterinary medical textbooks. More recent studies have linked the depression scoring in calves with increased

D-lactate concentrations instead of the severity of acidosis.[43,47] The clinical signs of increased D-lactate concentrations and their relationship to predicting academia in calves are described in the article by Lorenz and colleagues elsewhere in this issue.

In summary, the age of the calf needs to be taken into consideration when assessing the severity of acidosis and determining bicarbonate requirements of diarrheic calves. Calves with diarrhea and dehydration during their first week of life are less acidotic than older calves, and require less sodium bicarbonate to correct their acidemia. Calves that are unable to stand or that have a weak or absent suckle reflex have more severe acidosis and require IV sodium bicarbonate to correct their acidemia. D-Lactic acidosis may be present in sick calves with or without diarrhea and dehydration that are recumbent or wobbly; tired, listless or comatose; and with a delayed, incomplete, or absent palpebral reflex.[48] Also, if the suckle reflex is absent, weak, or the calf is chewing irregularly instead of suckling normal, D-lactic acidosis may be the underlying disease state.

Solutions for IV Administration

Thorough reviews of fluid therapy in ruminants and options for fluid therapy in calves with diarrhea have been published previously.[38,49,50] A brief overview of IV fluid therapy in calves is given here, with the focus primarily on more recent advances in the treatment of diarrhea. Because acidemia is common in calves with diarrhea, these animals generally require an alkalinizing fluid type to increase their blood pH. These fluids can include:

Lactated Ringer solution

Lactated Ringer solution (LRS) is a traditional isotonic fluid that is sometimes used to correct dehydration and electrolyte abnormalities in neonatal ruminants. Lactate is a metabolizable base and therefore LRS is considered an alkalinizing fluid (that can increase blood pH). However, because the lactate must be metabolized to produce an alkalinizing effect, this fluid type is considered to have weak or slow alkalinizing ability and is not recommended for neonates with severe acidemia.[24,31] Although LRS can successfully be used to treat dehydration and electrolyte abnormalities in neonates, it is difficult and expensive to administer in the field, requiring IV catheterization, delivery equipment, animal restraint, large fluid volumes (3–5 L in a calf depending on size and degree of dehydration), and monitoring. A theoretic disadvantage of commercially available LRS is that the lactate is a racemic equimolar mixture of L-lactate and D-lactate and its use should be avoided in severely acidemic calves because D-lactate concentrations may already be increased.[43,47]

Acetated Ringer solution

Acetated Ringer solution is similar to LRS but contains acetate instead of lactate as the metabolizable base. It is also considered a weak or slow alkalinizing fluid type and should be given in large volumes to correct dehydration in diarrheic calves. Acetated Ringer solution is theoretically superior to LRS because acetate is metabolized faster, therefore alkalinization is more rapid. In addition, acetate does not exacerbate the D-lactic acidosis present in most calves with diarrhea.

Isotonic sodium bicarbonate

Sodium bicarbonate is often referred to as a strong alkalinizing fluid because bicarbonate does not have to be metabolized by the liver to have an alkalinizing effect on the blood. Sodium bicarbonate has proved to be more effective than other metabolizable bases (such as lactate or acetate), bicarbonate precursors, or synthetic bases.[31,41] Isotonic sodium bicarbonate is often given as a 1.3% solution and can easily be prepared by adding baking soda ($NaHCO_3^-$) to sterile (or distilled) water at 13 g per liter (155 mEq/L HCO_3^-) and administered via an IV catheter. Isotonic sodium bicarbonate has an effective SID of 155 mEq/L and is alkalinizing because it buffers hydrogen ions and increases the SID in blood. The amount of isotonic bicarbonate required to correct an acidemia is usually calculated based on either blood total CO_2 or bicarbonate concentrations, or base excess values, but usually ranges between 2 and 5 L depending on the calf's weight and severity of acidosis (which can be estimated using depression scores). Base excess values calculated from blood gas analysis or estimated from depression scoring charts are multiplied by body weight, and with a factor that considers the volume of distribution for bicarbonate ions in the body (generally 0.6) according to the following formula:

Bicarbonate requirement (mEq) = body weight (kg) × base deficit (mEq/L) × 0.6 (L/kg)

Another simple but successful rule of thumb is to administer isotonic sodium bicarbonate solution at approximately 10% body weight over a period of several hours (eg, 4 L to a 40-kg calf). The disadvantage of isotonic sodium bicarbonate is that it requires an IV catheter and the administration of a large volume of fluids, which can sometimes be difficult to accomplish under field conditions.

Hypertonic saline
Over the past 10 years it has been discovered that hypertonic saline (2400 mOsm/L) can be used to rapidly expand plasma volume in a severely dehydrated calf.[51–53] When combined with oral electrolyte solutions, this therapy can be as effective in resuscitating severely dehydrated calves as large-volume LRS administration and is less expensive and much easier to administer. Hypertonic saline solutions can be purchased commercially in 1000-mL containers and should be given at a rate of 4 to 5 mL/kg administered slowly over a 4-minute period. However, hypertonic saline does not correct an acidemia. Hypertonic saline is also indicated for the treatment of hyperkalemia in calves. It is effective in rapidly decreasing serum potassium concentrations and reversing electrocardiographic abnormalities associated with hyperkalemia.[54] This effect is likely caused by intracellular movement of potassium and extracellular volume expansion.

Hypertonic sodium bicarbonate
In recent years, the use of hypertonic sodium bicarbonate (HSB) combined with oral electrolytes has gained popularity for the correction of acidosis and dehydration in neonatal ruminants with diarrhea. In general, HSB is commercially available as an 8.4% solution that contains sodium bicarbonate at 1 mEq/mL of solution (**Fig. 2**). The total osmolality is approximately 2000 mOsm/L. Therefore the product should theoretically generate an osmotic movement of water and electrolytes from the gastrointestinal tract to the ECF space similar to hypertonic saline. However, an added benefit is that it is an alkalinizing fluid and should significantly increase blood pH at the same time. Although there are some theoretic disadvantages to HSB administration, a study in anesthetized calves showed that rapid administration of HSB was safe when administered to anesthetized calves.[55] It was effective in reversing an experimentally induced acidemia and did not cause cerebrospinal fluid pH to decrease (paradoxic cerebrospinal fluid acidosis) as has long been hypothesized. Other recent studies have also been done using HSB in calves with diarrhea. In a German study, 28 calves with naturally occurring diarrhea were divided into 2 groups.[46] One group received hypertonic saline (5 mL/kg of body weight over 4 minutes) and the other group received hypertonic (8.4%) sodium bicarbonate (10 mL/kg of body weight over 10 minutes).

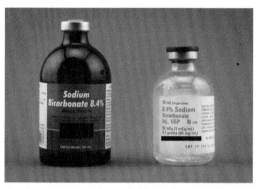

Fig. 2. Examples of 8.4% HSB commonly available in the United States. In North America, this product is typically sold in 100-mL bottles.

IV fluids were followed by 3 L of an isotonic oral electrolyte solution. During the 72-hour period following treatment, more calves recovered that had received the HSB compared with hypertonic saline (many calves that received only hypertonic saline required additional fluid therapy). Another study done in Turkey involved 50 calves with diarrhea, dehydration, and strong ion acidosis.[56] Thirty calves in this study received isotonic sodium bicarbonate (65 mL/kg of body weight over 3 hours), whereas 20 calves received 8.4% HSB (10 mL/kg of body weight over 20 minutes). No oral electrolytes were given to either group. Although isotonic sodium bicarbonate was able to increase plasma volume to a greater extent than HSB, both fluid types were effective in rapidly increasing venous pH and resuscitating calves. Although more studies are needed to determine the proper dose of HSB for use in calves, this can be an effective fluid type for correcting metabolic acidosis. It can be used in calves with diarrhea when an IV catheter or long-term fluid therapy is not practical. However, HSB should probably not be used in diarrheic calves that have concurrent respiratory disease, because these calves may not be able to effectively exhale the excess CO_2 generated in buffer reactions.

Dextrose

This is the only nonalkalinizing fluid type that is generally used in neonatal ruminants. Dextrose is often added to other solutions at 5% to 10% to counteract the negative energy balance in diarrheic calves with or without hypoglycemia. However, in dehydrated calves a plain 5% dextrose solution is not sufficient to correct ECF deficits because the solution contains no sodium. To provide energy and rehydrate the neonate, 25 to 50 g of dextrose or 50 to 100 mL of 50% dextrose solution can be added per liter of LRS or isotonic sodium bicarbonate to make a mildly hypertonic solution.

In summary, alkalinizing fluids are the appropriate choice for the IV rehydration of calves with diarrhea and dehydration. At present, sodium bicarbonate is the recommended solution for IV treatment of diarrheic calves that have lost their suckle reflex and palpebral reflex and are unwilling to stand. Sodium bicarbonate (either hypertonic or isotonic) rapidly corrects both acidosis and dehydration, and restores normal cellular function. When the calf's suckle reflex is reestablished, further treatment can be given orally.

ADMINISTRATION OF IV FLUIDS

Many studies have presented various protocols for IV fluid therapy in calves, but clinical research comparing the effectiveness of different protocols in dehydrated calves with diarrhea is limited. In practice, fluid therapy has to be simple and cost-effective, and must be based on clinical signs that are easily assessed. To determine daily fluid requirements, estimated amounts for replacement, maintenance, and ongoing losses (for diarrhea) must be calculated. The quantity of replacement fluid in liters is calculated by multiplying the estimated dehydration in percent with body weight in kilograms according to the following formula:

Replacement fluid (L) = dehydration (%) × body weight (kg)

A maximum rate of 80 mL/kg/h for IV fluid administration has been used without inducing significant overhydration and hypertension. This rate is equivalent to a maximum fluid volume of 2.8 L per hour for a 35-kg (77 lb) calf, or 3.8 L (1 gallon) per hour for a 47-kg (104 lb) severely dehydrated calf. Higher flow rates are not recommended. Slower infusion rates of 30 to 50 mL/kg/h are often used to avoid overhydration and pulmonary edema.[57] With a rate of 30 to 40 mL/kg/h, a 40-kg calf with 10% dehydration can be rehydrated within 3 to 4 hours. In addition, daily maintenance fluid volumes of 80 to 100 mL/kg and ongoing losses of up to 7 L per day should be added to calculate the daily fluid requirements. However, if the calf can suckle after initial resuscitation, these fluid requirements can be given orally to reduce costs. IV fluids are generally given via jugular or auricular (ear) vein catheter. Catheterization of the auricular vein in calves has been described in detail previously.[38]

As stated earlier, practitioners must rely on clinical signs such as ability to stand, suckling intensity, loss of palpebral reflex, and age of diarrheic calves to determine whether alkalinizing therapy is indicated and how much isotonic sodium bicarbonate should be administered. Because determining the severity of acidosis on the farm is difficult and costly, buffer administration is commonly done without any laboratory data. Therefore the clinical response of the calf to IV fluid therapy must be monitored. Urination within 30 to 60 minutes; improvement of mental and hydration status; and, most importantly, restoration of the suckle reflex are monitored as responses to treatment. Recumbent calves should stand within a few hours of IV fluid therapy. If the suckle reflex does not return after IV buffer therapy, other diseases such as septicemia, omphalitis, or pneumonia should be ruled out.

A Simplified Protocol for On-farm IV Fluid Therapy

A simplified protocol for IV fluid therapy using only 5-L bags of normal saline and 8.4% HSB has been used successfully in practice. Calves are examined for dehydration by evaluating the eyeball position within the orbit; for weakness and ability to stand by careful manipulation (not performed in comatose calves); for duration of anorexia by obtaining history and determining suckle reflex; and for hypothermia by palpation of extremities, oral cavity, and obtaining rectal temperature.

The standard treatment protocol for IV fluid therapy consists of a 5-L bag of isotonic saline (0.9% NaCl) to which 250 mL of 8.4% HSB (total of 250 mEq HCO_3^-) is added (**Fig. 3**), which creates a slightly hypertonic solution and is recommended for use in calves less than 1 week of age. All solutions are commercially available, and isotonic saline solution is supplied in plastic bags that are easily attachable in the calf's environment (**Fig. 4**). This protocol has also been used successfully in haul-in practices that do not have hospitalization facilities. The calf can be catheterized and the fluids hung on the wall inside the trailer. The calf's legs are tied together and then released when the 5-L bag of fluids has finished and the calf has returned to the farm. Calves presented with relapses after administration of this standard protocol receive another treatment when they are not able to suckle after the first treatment. Calves that fail to

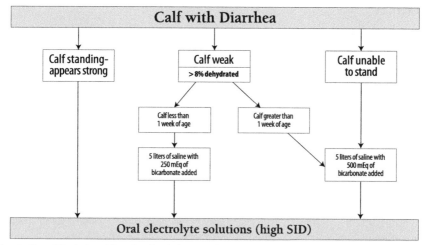

Fig. 3. Simplified algorithm for fluid therapy for dehydrated calves. This approach requires that the practitioner carry only 5-L bags of 0.9% saline and 8.4% HSB, which contains 1 mEq of bicarbonate per milliliter (thus, a 100-mL bottle equals 100 mEq of bicarbonate).

significantly improve in attitude, have a weak or absent suckle reflex, or show consistent weakness after 1 or 2 administrations of the standard (5 L) IV fluid solution are generally suspected of having a more severe acidosis. These calves then receive fluids containing a larger amount of sodium bicarbonate, especially when they are older than 1 week of age. Up to 750 mL of 8.4% sodium bicarbonate (750 mEq HCO_3^-) can be added to the 5-L bag of isotonic saline. Similar simplified protocols or decision trees for treating acidosis in calves with diarrhea have been published.[58]

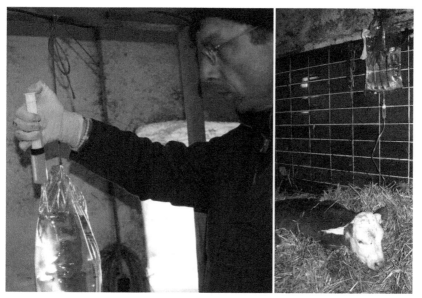

Fig. 4. Simplified protocol for fluid therapy in calves with diarrhea. HSB is added to 5-L bags of saline, which can be administered to calves over a period of 4 to 5 hours.

REFERENCES

1. Foster DM, Smith GW. Pathophysiology of diarrhea in calves. Vet Clin North Am Food Anim Pract 2009;25:13–36.
2. Smith GW. Treatment of calf diarrhea: oral fluid therapy. Vet Clin North Am Food Anim Pract 2009;25:55–72.
3. Michell AR. Drips, drinks and drenches: what matters in fluid therapy. Ir Vet J 1988;42:17–22.
4. Michell AR, Brooks HW, White DG, et al. The comparative effectiveness of three commercial oral solutions in correcting fluid, electrolyte and acid-base disturbances caused by calf diarrhoea. Br Vet J 1992;148:507–22.
5. Sen I, Constable PD, Marshall TS. Effect of suckling isotonic or hypertonic solutions of sodium bicarbonate or glucose on abomasal emptying rate in calves. Am J Vet Res 2006;67:1377–84.
6. Constable PD, Stämpfli HR, Navetat H, et al. Use of a quantitative strong ion approach to determine the mechanism for acid-base abnormalities in sick calves with or without diarrhea. J Vet Intern Med 2005;19:581–9.
7. Lewis LD, Phillips RW. Water and electrolyte losses in neonatal calves with acute diarrhea. A complete balance study. Cornell Vet 1972;62:596–607.
8. Desjeux JF, Tannenbaum C, Tai YH, et al. Effects of sugars and amino acids on sodium movement across small intestine. Am J Dis Child 1977;131: 331–40.
9. Fisher RB. The absorption of water and some small solute molecules from the isolated small intestine of the rat. J Physiol 1955;130:655–64.
10. Deminge C, Remesy C, Chartier F, et al. Effect of acetate or chloride anions on intestinal absorption of water and solutes in the calf. Am J Vet Res 1981;42: 1356–9.
11. Demigne C, Remesy C, Chartier F, et al. Utilization of volatile fatty acids and improvement of fluid therapy for treatment of dehydration in diarrheic calves. Ann Rech Vet 1983;14:541–7.
12. Jodal M, Lundgren O. Countercurrent mechanisms in the mammalian intestinal tract. Gastroenterology 1986;91:225–41.
13. Levy M, Marritt AM, Levy LC. Comparison of the effects of an isosmolar and hyperosmolar oral rehydrating solution on the hydration status, glycemia and ileal content composition of healthy neonatal calves. Cornell Vet 1990;80: 143–51.
14. Constable PD, Thomas E, Boisrame B. Comparison of two oral electrolyte solutions for the treatment of dehydrated calves with experimentally-induced diarrhea. Vet J 2001;162:129–40.
15. Brooks HW, White DG, Wagstaff AJ, et al. Evaluation of a nutritive oral rehydration solution for the treatment of calf diarrhoea. Br Vet J 1996;152:699–708.
16. Fettman MJ, Brooks PA, Burrows KP, et al. Evaluation of commercial oral replacement formulas in healthy neonatal calves. J Am Vet Med Assoc 1986; 188:397–401.
17. Sen I, Altunok V, Ok M, et al. Efficacy of oral rehydration therapy solutions containing sodium bicarbonate or sodium acetate for treatment of calves with naturally acquired diarrhea, moderate dehydration, and strong ion acidosis. J Am Vet Med Assoc 2009;234:926–34.
18. Nouri M, Constable PD. Comparison of two oral electrolyte solutions and route of administration on the abomasal emptying rate of Holstein-Friesian calves. J Vet Intern Med 2006;20:620–6.

19. Panciera RJ, Boileau MJ, Step DL. Tympany, acidosis, and mural emphysema of the stomach in calves: report of cases and experimental induction. J Vet Diagn Invest 2007;19:392–5.
20. Songer JG, Miskimins DW. Clostridial abomasitis in calves: case report and review of the literature. Anaerobe 2005;11:290–4.
21. Marshall TS. Abomasal ulceration and tympany of calves. Vet Clin North Am Food Anim Pract 2009;25:209–20.
22. Groutides CP, Michell AR. Changes in plasma composition in calves surviving or dying from diarrhoea. Br Vet J 1990;146:205–10.
23. Tennant B, Harrold D, Reina-Guerra M. Physiologic and metabolic factors in the pathogenesis of neonatal enteric infections in calves. J Am Vet Med Assoc 1972;161:993–1007.
24. Kasari TR, Naylor JM. Clinical evaluation of sodium bicarbonate, sodium L-lactate, and sodium acetate for the treatment of acidosis in diarrheic calves. J Am Vet Med Assoc 1985;187:392–7.
25. Smith GW, Ahmed AF, Constable PD. Effect of orally administered electrolyte solution formulation on abomasal luminal pH and emptying rate in dairy calves. J Am Vet Med Assoc 2012;241:1075–82.
26. Bachmann L, Homeier T, Arlt S. Influence of different oral rehydration solutions on abomasal conditions and the acid-base status of suckling calves. J Dairy Sci 2009;92:1649–59.
27. Marshall TS, Constable PD, Crochik SS, et al. Effect of suckling an isotonic solution of sodium acetate, sodium bicarbonate, or sodium chloride on abomasal emptying rate and luminal pH in calves. Am J Vet Res 2008;69:824–31.
28. Martinsen TC, Bergh K, Waldum HL. Gastric juice: a barrier against infectious diseases. Basic Clin Pharmacol Toxicol 2005;96:94–102.
29. Wray C, Callow RJ. Studies on the survival of Salmonella dublin, S. typhimurium, and E. coli in stored bovine colostrum. Vet Rec 1974;94:407–12.
30. Zhu H, Hart CA, Sales D, et al. Bacterial killing in gastric juice – effect of pH and pepsin on Escherichia coli and Helicobacter pylori. J Med Microbiol 2006;55:1265–70.
31. Naylor JM, Forsyth GW. The alkalinizing effects of metabolizable bases in the healthy calf. Can J Vet Res 1986;50:509–16.
32. Naylor JM, Petrie L, Rodriguez MI, et al. A comparison of three oral electrolyte solutions in the treatment of diarrheic calves. Can Vet J 1990;31:753–60.
33. Booth AJ, Naylor JM. Correction of metabolic acidosis in diarrheal calves by oral administration of electrolyte solutions with or without bicarbonate. J Am Vet Med Assoc 1987;191:62–8.
34. Stämpfli H, Oliver O, Pringle JK. Clinical evaluation of an oral electrolyte solution formulated based on strong ion difference (SID) and using propionate as the organic anion in the treatment of neonatal diarrheic calves with strong ion acidosis. Open J Vet Med 2012;2:34–9.
35. Dupe RJ, Goddard ME, Bywater RJ. A comparison of two oral rehydration solutions in experimental models of dehydration and diarrhoea in calves. Vet Rec 1989;125:620–4.
36. Garthwaite BD, Drackley JK, McCoy GC, et al. Whole milk and oral rehydration solution for calves with diarrhea of spontaneous origin. J Dairy Sci 1994;77:835–43.
37. Goodell GM, Campbell J, Hoejvang-Nielsen L, et al. An alkalinizing oral rehydration solution containing lecithin-coated citrus fiber is superior to a nonalkalinizing solution in treating 360 calves with naturally acquired diarrhea. J Dairy Sci 2012;95:6677–86.

38. Berchtold J. Treatment of calf diarrhea: intravenous fluid therapy. Vet Clin North Am Food Anim Pract 2009;25:73–100.
39. Constable PD, Walker PG, Morin DE, et al. Use of peripheral temperature and core-temperature difference to predict cardiac output in dehydrated calves housed in a thermoneutral environment. Am J Vet Res 1998;59:874–80.
40. Kasari TR, Naylor JM. Further studies on the clinical features and clinicopathological findings of a syndrome of metabolic acidosis with minimal or no dehydration in neonatal calves. Can J Vet Res 1986;50:502–8.
41. Naylor JM. Severity and nature of acidosis in diarrheic calves over and under one week of age. Can Vet J 1987;28:168–73.
42. Naylor JM. A retrospective study of the relationship between clinical signs and severity of acidosis in diarrheic calves. Can Vet J 1989;30:577–80.
43. Lorenz I. Influence of D-lactate on metabolic acidosis and on prognosis in neonatal calves with diarrhoea. J Vet Med A Physiol Pathol Clin Med 2004;51: 425–8.
44. Grove-White DH, White DG. Diagnosis and treatment of metabolic acidosis in calves: a field study. Vet Rec 1993;133:499–501.
45. Grove-White D, Michell AR. Comparison of the measurement of total carbon dioxide and strong ion difference for the evaluation of metabolic acidosis in diarrhoeic calves. Vet Rec 2001;148:365–70.
46. Koch A, Kaske M. Clinical efficacy of intravenous hypertonic saline solution or hypertonic bicarbonate solution in the treatment of inappetent calves with neonatal diarrhea. J Vet Intern Med 2008;22:202–11.
47. Lorenz I, Vogt S. Investigations on the association of D-lactate blood concentration with the outcome of therapy of acidosis, and with posture and demeanor in young calves with diarrhoea. J Vet Med A Physiol Pathol Clin Med 2006;53: 490–4.
48. Trefz FM, Lorch A, Feist M, et al. Metabolic acidosis in neonatal calf diarrhea – clinical findings and theoretical assessment of a simple treatment protocol. J Vet Intern Med 2012;26:162–70.
49. Constable PD. Fluid and electrolyte therapy in ruminants. Vet Clin North Am Food Anim Pract 2003;19:557–97.
50. Berchtold J. Intravenous fluid therapy of calves. Vet Clin North Am Food Anim Pract 1999;15:505–31.
51. Constable PD, Schmall LM, Muir WW III, et al. Hemodynamic response of endotoxemic calves to treatment with small-volume hypertonic saline solution. Am J Vet Res 1991;52:981–9.
52. Walker PG, Constable PD, Morin DE, et al. Comparison of hypertonic saline-dextran solution and lactated Ringer's solution for resuscitating severely dehydrated calves with diarrhea. J Am Vet Med Assoc 1998;213:113–21.
53. Leal ML, Fialho SS, Cyrillo FC, et al. Intravenous hypertonic saline solution (7.5%) and oral electrolytes to treat calves with noninfectious diarrhea and metabolic acidosis. J Vet Intern Med 2012;26:1042–50.
54. Constable PD. Hypertonic saline. Vet Clin North Am Food Anim Pract 1999;15: 559–85.
55. Berchtold JP, Constable PD, Smith GW, et al. Effects of intravenous hyperosmotic sodium bicarbonate on arterial and cerebrospinal fluid acid-base status and cardiovascular function in calves with experimentally induced respiratory and strong ion acidosis. J Vet Intern Med 2005;19:240–51.
56. Coskun A, Sen I, Guzelbektes J, et al. Comparison of the effects of intravenous administration of isotonic and hypertonic sodium bicarbonate solutions on

venous acid-base status in dehydrated calves with strong ion acidosis. J Am Vet Med Assoc 2010;236:1098–103.

57. Roussel AJ. Principles and mechanics of fluid therapy in calves. Compend Cont Educ Pract Vet 1983;5:S332–6.

58. Trefz FM, Lorch A, Feist M, et al. Construction and validation of a decision tree for treating metabolic acidosis in calves with neonatal diarrhea. BMC Vet Res 2012;8:238.

Fluid Therapy in Mature Cattle

Allen J. Roussel, DVM, MS

KEYWORDS

- Electrolytes • Fluid therapy • Cattle • Acidosis • Alkalosis • Hypokalemia
- Hypochloremia

KEY POINTS

- Fluid therapy for mature cattle differs from that of calves because the common conditions that result in dehydration and the metabolic derangements that accompany these conditions are different.
- The veterinarian needs to know the problem which exists, what to administer to correct the problem, in what quantity, by what route and at what rate.
- Mature cattle more frequently suffer from alkalosis, therefore acidifying solutions containing K^+ and Cl^- in concentrations greater than that of plasma are frequently indicated.
- While intravenous therapy is critical to some patients, seldom does the entire deficit need to be administered intravenously.
- The rumen provides a large-capacity reservoir into which oral rehydration solutions may be administered, which can save time and money.

INTRODUCTION

It might be surprising to some that we've chosen to discuss fluid therapy of mature cattle apart from calves in this issue. Although there are some minor differences in technique and strategy owing to size and logistical considerations, and because mature cattle have a rumen, these are not the most important reasons to divide the discussion. Mostly when fluid therapy is administered to cattle the choice of solution, route, and so forth is based on empirical data such as signalment, history, clinical signs, and diagnosis of the primary problem. Because the most common causes of dehydration or shock, and their resulting metabolic and electrolyte derangements, differ between mature cattle and calves, the rehydration solution appropriate for most dehydrated calves is not the most appropriate solution for most dehydrated mature cattle. Therefore, it makes sense to discuss these 2 classes of cattle separately.

The author has no conflicts to disclose.
Department of Large Animal Clinical Sciences, College of Veterinary Medicine and Biomedical Sciences, Texas A&M University, 4475 TAMU, College Station, TX 77843-4475, USA
E-mail address: aroussel@cvm.tamu.edu

The approach to fluid, electrolyte, and acid-base therapy occasionally becomes complicated by tables, charts, and formulas. Although these tools are essential for the complete understanding of principles and mechanisms, the clinical approach to fluid therapy simply requires the clinician to answer 4 questions. (1) What is the problem? (2) What solution do I administer to correct the problem? (3) How much do I administer? (4) By what route and at what rate should I administer the solution?

WHAT IS THE PROBLEM?

This question is really asking "what are the metabolic derangements in the electrolyte and acid-base status of the animal being treated?" When the definitive diagnosis is known and laboratory data are available, the answer to this question is simple and specific. For most cases, however, the veterinarian does not have the advantage of all of these data. Therefore, assumptions of these problems are made based on clinical signs and presumptive or definitive diagnosis.

Dehydration

The most frequent indication for fluid therapy in mature cattle is dehydration. In some instances, shock without substantial dehydration might occur. Shock might occur secondarily to iatrogenic or accidental hemorrhage or acute endotoxemia. Shock can be identified by a rapid heart rate, pale mucous membranes, delayed capillary refill time, and weakness or collapse. Capillary refill time is more difficult to assess in cattle than in horses and small animals. In some animals, the vulva may be a more reliable site than the oral mucous membranes. Capillary refill time of greater than 2 seconds suggests shock.

Dehydration may occur with or without accompanying shock, and is indicated by eyeball recession into the sockets, increased skin turgor, and dry or tacky oral mucous membranes. Eyeball recession is assessed by pulling the lower eyelid ventrally with the fingers to determine if there is a gap between the globe and the orbit. A gap indicates dehydration. One must be aware, however, that eyeball recession also occurs in emaciation. Therefore, very thin cows should be assessed using multiple clinical signs for hydration status. In older bulls and *Bos indicus* cattle, the skin of the neck can be fairly thick, making assessment of skin turgor difficult. Tenting the skin and measuring the time it takes to return to its normal position after release is used to determine skin turgor. Typically, longer than 2 to 3 seconds is considered delayed and suggests clinical dehydration.

Acidosis or Alkalosis?

Another fundamental consideration when approaching fluid therapy is that of acid-base status. Ideally, blood gas analysis including the base excess (BE) is used establish a diagnosis and guide therapy. A negative BE indicates metabolic acidosis and a positive BE indicates metabolic alkalosis. When blood gas analysis is not available, the measurement of serum bicarbonate (HCO_3^-) or total carbon dioxide (TCO_2) can substitute as an indicator of metabolic acid-base status. Plasma HCO_3^- and TCO_2 are decreased in acidosis and increased in alkalosis. When laboratory data are not available, the clinician can make assumptions about the acid-base status of mature cattle based on clinical signs or diagnosis. It is well documented that, unlike calves, most mature cattle with dehydration are not acidotic. Therefore, therapy aimed at correcting acidosis is not indicated. In a study of more than 500 cattle older than 1 month, blood gas and electrolyte determinations were made from venous blood samples.[1] Dehydrated mature cattle were about twice as likely to have metabolic alkalosis than metabolic acidosis. If cattle with pneumonia, carbohydrate engorgement (rumen acidosis), and diarrhea were excluded, only 16% of dehydrated cattle had metabolic acidosis. In another study, approximately 60% of 350 sick cattle tested had pH values within the reference interval.[2] However, many had compensated acidosis or alkalosis. Approximately 53% had abnormally elevated concentrations of HCO_3^-, whereas about 10% had decreased HCO_3^- concentrations. Therefore, based simply on the fact that an animal is a mature bovid and is dehydrated, the probability that it has metabolic alkalosis is much greater than the probability that it has metabolic acidosis. By considering the clinical signs and diagnosis, further refinement of the assumption can be made. Gastrointestinal tract stasis and small intestinal or pyloric obstruction lead to accumulation of chloride ions in the gastrointestinal tract, resulting in systemic alkalosis. Therefore, cattle with abomasal displacement or volvulus, vagal indigestion, and cecal displacement or torsion are usually alkalotic. Carbohydrate engorgement,[1] urinary tract disease,[1] small intestinal strangulation/obstruction,[2] and enteritis/diarrhea[1,2] are conditions of mature cattle whereby metabolic acidosis is more common than metabolic alkalosis. Carbohydrate engorgement results in systemic acidosis because large amounts of volatile fatty acids and lactic acid are produced by bacterial fermentation. Both D- and L-lactic acid are produced, but only the L-isomer is efficiently metabolized by mammalian tissues. Choke or other causes of salivary loss are also causes of acidosis because ruminant saliva is rich in sodium bicarbonate. Relatively common diseases that are inconsistent but potential causes of serious acidosis include diarrhea, fatty liver disease, and urinary tract disease.[1–3] Cattle and small ruminants with urethral obstruction or uroperitoneum usually do not have clinically important changes in acid-base status. In a study of 108 goats with urolithiasis, 44.8% had mild to moderate metabolic alkalosis while 10% had mild metabolic acidosis.[4] Some diseases usually associated with alkalosis may be accompanied by acidosis in the later stages of the disease; these include abomasal volvulus, intussusception, and torsion of the mesenteric root.[2,5]

Electrolyte Abnormalities

In addition to acid-base imbalances, the derangements of plasma electrolytes are frequent in mature cattle. In the aforementioned study, approximately 20% of dehydrated cattle were hyponatremic or hypokalemic while more than 40% were hypochloremic.[1] Hypochloridemia and hypokalemia frequently accompany metabolic alkalosis in cattle.[2,3,6,7] Approximately 50% of postpartum dairy cows fed a typical diet developed hypocalcemia.[8]

Hypernatremia, hyperkalemia, and hyperchloremia are relatively rare conditions, occurring in 11%, 11%, and 16%, respectively, of dehydrated cattle in one large study.[1] Hypernatremia in mature cattle is almost always associated with water restriction or salt intoxication, is usually accompanied by hyperchloremia, and is frequently associated with depression or neurologic signs. Hyperkalemia occurs secondarily to metabolic acidosis in mature cattle, as in calves. Unlike monogastrics, ruminants do not typically develop hyperkalemia with obstructive urolithiasis or urinary tract rupture.[4,9,10] Hyperkalemia developed in only 16.8% of goats with urolithiasis and in fewer than 50% of those with urinary tract rupture. None of the elevations were life-threatening.[4]

WHAT DO I ADMINISTER TO CORRECT THE PROBLEM?
Dehydration

The obvious solution to the problem of dehydration might seem to be water, and although water is absolutely essential to correct dehydration, it is not sufficient. As discussed in the previous section, dehydrated cattle are infrequently hyperosmolar. Most of the water loss is either iso-osmotic or hyperosmotic, resulting in a dehydrated animal that requires not only water but also electrolytes to repair its extracellular fluid disturbance. For this reason, free water (administered in the form of 5% dextrose) is seldom an appropriate rehydration fluid. Rather, for replacement, electrolytes must be administered along with water in concentrations similar to or greater than that found in plasma. For maintenance, solutions that contain physiologic concentrations of sodium and chloride with additional potassium are usually most appropriate. Additional potassium is required because potassium is continually excreted in the urine, and also because many cattle requiring fluid therapy are anorectic and therefore are not taking in adequate amounts of potassium to maintain homeostasis. Additional calcium is also frequently required, particularly in postpartum dairy cows.

Acid-Base Balance and Electrolytes

One of the first critical decisions to be made in selecting an appropriate solution for administration is whether the solution should be alkalinizing or not. If appropriate laboratory equipment is available, it is relatively simple to determine if solutions should be alkalinizing by performing a blood gas analysis or evaluating plasma TCO_2 concentration. As discussed previously, acidosis is not a common occurrence in dehydrated mature cattle. When it does occur, it is corrected just as in calves. Merely restoring extracellular fluid volume was not sufficient to rapidly correct acidosis in diarrheic calves.[11] Because it is preferable to correct the metabolic abnormalities of cattle quickly for convenience and cost savings, it is usually recommended that alkalinizing agents be included in rehydration fluids for acidotic cattle. Alkalinizing solutions contain bicarbonate or metabolizable bases that result in the consumption on a hydrogen ion (or increase in the strong ion difference) when metabolized. Sodium bicarbonate is the most economical and readily available alkalinizing agent. However, it cannot be heat sterilized and ideally should not be used in solutions containing calcium, as an insoluble compound will be formed.

Alternative alkalinizing agents offer advantages and disadvantages. Lactate is probably the most widely used alkalinizing agent in veterinary medicine in the United States. Commercial preparations of lactated Ringer solution contain racemic mixtures of D- and L-lactate. Only the L-isomer is metabolized efficiently (by Lorenz and colleagues elsewhere in this issue for further information). Therefore, the alkalinizing potential of the racemic mixture is less than the total amount of lactate in the solution. Unlike lactate, acetate is metabolized by peripheral tissues, not just the liver. It has no significant endogenous source and no nonmetabolized isomer. Gluconate, an alkalinizing agent used in combination with acetate in commercially prepared solutions for intravenous administration to humans, dogs, and horses, has been shown to be ineffective as an alkalinizing agent in calves.[12] Dire warnings about the dangers of rapid administration of sodium bicarbonate solution are widespread in the veterinary and medical literature, but appear to be unfounded in cattle practice. Much anecdotal experience and a recent research report suggest that rapid correction of acidosis in cattle is usually without the complication of cerebrospinal fluid acidosis.[13]

When blood pH and TCO_2 are within the reference interval, balanced solutions such as lactated Ringer with additional potassium chloride and calcium may be administered. Alternatively, 0.9% NaCl with K and Ca may be used. Even though lactated Ringer solution may have a tendency to alkalinize an animal and 0.9% NaCl may have a tendency to acidify an animal, the use of these solutions to rehydrate an animal with normal acid-base balance is unlikely to create a significant metabolic imbalance.

When significant alkalosis is present, one should choose an acidifying solution that contains K^+ and Cl^- in excess of physiologic concentrations. The acidifying properties of a high K^+ and Cl^- solution can be explained using the principles of strong ion difference theory. In brief, increasing the relative amount of strong anions, in this case Cl^-, in the plasma reduces strong ion difference and acidifies the extracellular fluid. Supplying part of the Cl^- as KCl enhances this effect because K^+ may move into the intracellular space or may be available for excretion in the kidneys, thus allowing renal compensation of alkalosis to proceed efficiently. For lactating cattle, the administration of calcium-containing solutions is recommended.

In the absence of laboratory analysis, assumptions of the acid-base balance should be made based on the clinical signs and presumptive diagnosis, as discussed earlier. Using simple probability, it is much less likely that a dehydrated bovid requires correction of the metabolic acidosis than correction of metabolic alkalosis. In cattle with little nutritional intake, lactating cattle, or cattle in late gestation, the addition of glucose to rehydration fluids is important.

HOW MUCH DO I ADMINISTER?
Volume

Constable and colleagues[14] showed that the time required for cervical skin to return to its normal position after tenting and the degree of eyeball recession in dehydrated preruminant calves are reasonably accurate methods to determine the state of hydration for calves. For example, when skin pinched on the neck takes 6 seconds to return to normal, this indicates 8% dehydration (**Table 1**). There have not been similar quantitative studies of the relationship between clinical signs and degree of dehydration for mature ruminants. In the absence of data to suggest otherwise, the values for estimating dehydration in calves using a skin tent is probably a reasonable guide for mature cattle. However, emaciation can cause eyeball recession and loss of skin turgor, making these tests more difficult to interpret in cattle that have recently lost substantial body condition. The body weight of mature ruminants can change dramatically based on the amount of ingesta and water in the rumen, so estimates of percent dehydration measured as a percentage of body weight are probably not very accurate. Therefore, from a clinical standpoint, it can be predicted that a cow which is 10% dehydrated will have a normal or near-normal hydration status if 10% of her body weight in fluids is restored. She may still be well under her "normal" body weight because of lack of rumen fill. On the other hand, a cow with forestomach distension from vagal indigestion or carbohydrate engorgement may gain weight from fluid sequestered in the third space compartment inside the rumen during the disease process, but may lose significant extracellular body water.

Rather than overemphasizing the need to exactly predict the quantity of rehydration fluids necessary to completely restore a cow to normal hydration status, one should focus on making a reasonable estimate of fluid deficit, then formulate an initial plan

Table 1								
Guide to the estimation of dehydration of calves using eyeball recession and skin tent								
% Dehydration	0	2	4	6	8	10	12	14
Eyeball recession (mm)	0	1	2	3	4	6	7	8
Skin-tent duration (s)	2	3	4	5	6	7	8	10

Data from Constable PD, Walker PG, Morin DE, et al. Clinical and laboratory assessment of hydration status of neonatal calves with diarrhea. J Am Vet Med Assoc 1998;212:991–6.

aimed at effecting clinical improvement. After initial therapy, further therapy can be adjusted as warranted by the patient's condition. This approach of "guess and reassess" is useful when treating large animals that require large quantities of fluids. One must bear in mind that, over 24 to 48 hours, not only must the fluid deficit be replaced but the animal must also be provided with sufficient water for maintenance, and replacement of ongoing water and electrolyte loss. Maintenance requirements for water depend on the ambient temperature and dry matter intake in addition to lactation. For nonlactating cattle at moderate ambient temperature, approximately 3.5% to 5% of body weight in water is required daily. Therefore, for a 500-kg animal, it will be necessary to provide 17.5% to 20% of body weight, or 88 to 100 L, over 48 hours. In addition, if ongoing losses are occurring, even more fluid must be provided. However, not all of this fluid must be administered intravenously. How to determine the appropriate route and rate of administration is discussed in a later section.

Correcting Acidosis

After the volume of fluid that must be replaced is determined, one must determine what goes into the solution. Calculating the total base required to correct acidosis is performed with a formula very similar to that used to calculate the amount required for the treatment of acidotic calves.

$$BD \times 0.3 \times BW \text{ (kg)} = \text{Total mEq of base required}$$

where BD is base deficit in mEq/L, 0.3 is a conversion factor for extracellular volume or the "bicarbonate space", and BW is body weight in kilograms. The base required is expressed as total mEq of base. Note that because extracellular water makes up a larger percentage of body weight in neonates than in mature cattle, the conversion factor 0.3 is used for mature cattle. This formula may represent an oversimplification of the correction of acid-base balance. A study in human patients suggests that as the plasma HCO_3 decreases the bicarbonate space increases, so that in severely acidotic animals this formula may underestimate the amount of base needed to correct the acidosis.[15] If the value for BE is not available, but that of TCO_2 or HCO_3 is available, the BD can be estimated using the formula

$$25 - TCO_2 \text{ (or } HCO_3) = BD$$

because 25 mEq/L represents the reference value for normal cattle. When laboratory data is not available, and there is a strong probability that moderate or severe acidosis exists, a BD of 10 mEq/L may be used without substantial risk as an estimate in the formula for initial therapy. If the cow in fact had a normal acid-base balance, creating a BE of 10 is unlikely to cause significant deterioration in the clinical status of the cow. If, instead, the cow had severe acidosis, improving the BE 10 mEq/L could improve the clinical status of the cow significantly. In theory, to move the BE by 10 mEq/L, the total base required for a 500-kg cow is:

$$10 \text{ mEq/L} \times 0.3 \times 500 \text{ kg} = 1500 \text{ mEq}$$

Sodium bicarbonate solution is marketed as a 5% (0.6 mEq/L) and 8.4% (1 mEq/L) solution in several container sizes, including 500 mL. In the author's experience, these products have been unavailable at certain times. Three 500-mL bottles of 8.4% $NaHCO_3$ provides 1500 mEq/L. if one wishes to formulate a nearly isotonic solution, one 500-mL bottle of 8.4% $NaHCO_3$ solution is added to 2500 mL of sterile water. It is also possible to use $NaHCO_3$ (baking soda) to formulate a fluid solution for intravenous administration. If hypertonic $NaHCO_3$ solutions are not available as described here, isotonic sodium bicarbonate can be prepared by adding 13 g of $NaHCO_3$ or baking soda to 1 L of sterile water. Each gram of baking soda has 12 mEq of HCO_3^-. Therefore, in the example discussed one would need to administer 125 g of baking soda to provide 1500 mEq of HCO_3^- to a 500-kg cow. At 13 g per liter, that would be equivalent to almost 10 L of isotonic $NaHCO_3$ to move the BE by 10 mEq/L. It may also be possible to administer hypertonic solutions of $NaHCO_3$ (for example, 125 g of baking soda dissolved in 5 L) when the administration of larger fluid volumes is not feasible.

Electrolytes

It is impossible to calculate the total body potassium deficit of an animal by measuring the plasma potassium because only about 5% of total body potassium is found in extracellular fluid. Instead, solutions are often empirically formulated with a concentration of 10 to 20 mEq/L of K^+. Considerably more is required for hypokalemic cattle (by Fecteau and colleagues elsewhere in this issue for further information). Because 1 g of KCl provides 14 mEq K^+, the addition of 1 to 2 g of KCl per liter of solution is a reasonable routine recommendation. Calcium may be added to solutions for intravenous administration. Ringer solution contains 5 mEq of calcium per liter and lactated Ringer contains 4 mEq/L. Inclusion of supplemental calcium is recommended in all fluids administered intravenously to lactating dairy cows unless calcium supplementation has been administered within the previous 12 hours. As a rule of thumb, 500 mL of a commercial calcium borogluconate solution may be added to 20 L of solution for intravenous administration. Alternatively, 10 g of calcium chloride may be substituted at a substantially lower cost.

BY WHAT ROUTE DO I ADMINISTER THE SOLUTIONS AND AT WHAT RATE?

Now that the composition and amount of the solution has been determined, only the route of administration and rate remain to be decided. Obviously the oral route will always be the most rapid and least expensive, and should be used as much as possible. However, in some cases intravenous therapy is the only reasonable choice. Somewhat arbitrarily, a cutoff of 8% dehydration has been proposed as the upper limit for choosing oral versus intravenous fluid therapy.[3,16] Even if the hydration status of a ruminant patient could be predicted with certainty, there are still factors other than hydration to consider when planning and executing the rehydration process. There are times when an experienced veterinarian can or must break the 8% rule. Sometimes cattle with severe dehydration and normal gastrointestinal function will recover uneventfully with only oral or intraruminal rehydration, or with a combination of intraruminal rehydration and a small amount of intravenously administered fluids. In these cases, breaking the rule saves substantial time and expense. On the other hand, endotoxemic or hypovolemic cattle may go into shock with only mild or moderate dehydration, and require intravenous fluids. Acute strangulating gastrointestinal disease and acute mastitis are examples of conditions that result in this situation. Rapidly correcting or preventing shock is particularly important if a standing surgical procedure is planned. This aspect is particularly important with volvuli or strangulating lesions of the gut where reperfusion of ischemic areas is critical. Finally, patients with fatty liver, chronic or refractory ketosis, and pregnancy toxemia may benefit from intravenous glucose therapy regardless of hydration status.

The idea of having to administer 100 L of rehydration solution intravenously might persuade one to abandon the idea of intravenous fluids completely. For this reason, it is critically important to remember that severely dehydrated cattle need some, but not all, fluids administered intravenously. For reasons no better than 20 L being the size of the container used to deliver intravenous fluids at his hospital, the author has rapidly administered only 20 to 40 L of intravenous fluid to many severely dehydrated cattle, with good results. If the underlying problem can be corrected, 20 to 40 L of intravenous fluids will often convert a severely dehydrated cow that requires intravenous therapy into a moderately or mildly dehydrated cow for which the residual dehydration can be corrected orally or intraruminally. One must not forget, however that, by one route or another, the animal needs to receive more than simply the calculated fluid deficit.

A flow rate of less than 80 mL/kg/h has been recommended for calves based on studies of central venous pressure in clinically dehydrated calves.[17] Similar studies have not been performed to determine the maximum safe flow rate in mature cattle or small ruminants. However, statistically significant elevations in central venous pressure occurred when approximately 40 mL/kg/h of an isotonic crystalloid solution was administered intravenously to dehydrated cattle with experimentally induced intestinal obstruction, even though no adverse clinical effects were observed.[18] Although this is a much slower flow rate than the maximal flow rate recommended for calves (80 mL/kg/h)[17] and dogs (90 mL/kg/h),[19] 40 mL/kg/h for an average dairy cow is a volume nearly impossible to achieve with a single 14-gauge intravenous catheter using gravity flow; this would represent 20 L/h for a 500-kg cow. Therefore, in most situations intravenous fluids can be safely administered to mature cattle through a 14-gauge catheter as quickly as they will flow by gravity. Exceptions include cattle with heart disease, oliguric renal failure, and hypoproteinemia, and those in recumbency.

A maximum flow rate of 0.5 mEq/kg BW per hour for potassium has been suggested for avoidance of fatal cardiac arrhythmias caused by hyperkalemia. If the solution contains 25 mEq/L, 20 mL contains 0.5 mEq K^+. Therefore the solution could be safely administered at a rate of 20 mL/kg/h, which is faster than the maximum flow rate through a 14-gauge catheter for most moderately and larger sized cattle. If 500 mL of 23% calcium borogluconate solution is added to 20 L of electrolyte solution, the infusion rate of the calcium should be well below the maximum safe flow rate.

Dextrose is frequently added to isotonic electrolyte solutions to make 2.5% to 5% dextrose solution. Rapid administration of glucose results in glucosuria, and may result in osmotic diuresis. There are no publications in the literature that demonstrate an optimal flow rate for intravenous administration of glucose to cattle. Several variables are involved in the regulation of blood glucose. Monitoring the excretion of glucose in the urine with dry chemistry sticks is a sensitive method, but perhaps is overly sensitive for adjusting the rate of glucose administration. When 500 mL of 50% dextrose solution was intravenously infused rapidly into cattle, less than 5% of the infused glucose was lost in urine. Nevertheless, glucose was detectable in the urine for 12 hours, suggesting that monitoring urine glucose may lead to the false impression that much glucose is being lost in the urine when, in fact, the vast majority is being retained.[20] Intravenous administration of glucose results in significant phosphaturia; therefore, cattle at risk of hypophosphatemia should be monitored carefully if glucose is administered intravenously.[20]

Techniques for Administration

A significant energy penalty is incurred if cold fluids are administered intravenously and must be warmed by the patient; therefore, warmed fluids should be administered.[21] Ideally, commercially prepared solutions should be used. However, optimal solutions for the abnormalities that occur in mature ruminants are not readily available in some countries. In such cases, sterilizing locally prepared fluids is recommended. All of the usual components of solutions for cattle can be heat sterilized, except sodium bicarbonate, which must be filtered. Alternatively, sterile distilled water and reagent-grade salts can be used to formulate solutions. Contamination should be carefully avoided during and after preparation, and solutions should be used immediately after preparation. Bacteria can be eliminated by autoclaving, but heat-stable endotoxins and pyrogens may be present in rural and municipal tap water.[22,23] Therefore, the use of pyrogen-free water is important.

The jugular vein is most frequently used for intravenous administration in adult cattle, and is the most useful for very rapid administration of large volumes. However, use of the auricular vein is fairly satisfactory for routine use (**Fig. 1**). This vein provides easy accessibility, is easy to place, and requires less expensive disposables. A 14-gauge catheter can usually be inserted in an auricular vein of a mature cow. Flow rates of greater than 7.5 L/h have been achieved with a 14-gauge catheter in the auricular vein. Auricular vein catheters have been maintained for longer than 96 hours with just twice-daily flushing with heparinized saline.[24]

The merit of hypertonic saline solution combined with intraruminal water or rehydration solution has been documented, and offers another option for rehydration. The usual dose is 4 to 5 mL of hypertonic saline (2400 mOsmol/L) solution per kilogram BW administered intravenously over 5 minutes and 20 L of water administered orally. Water should be pumped into the rumen of cattle treated with hypertonic saline if they

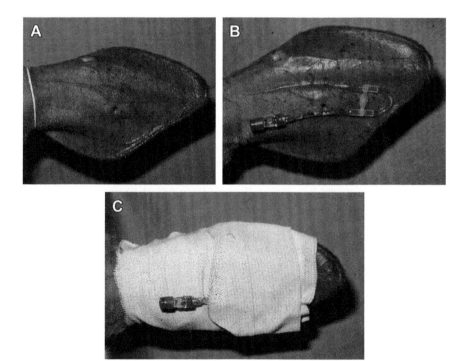

Fig. 1. (*A*) Proper site for placing auricular vein catheter in the ear of a cow. (*B*) Note that the vein is entered distally so that the tip will not kink at the base of the ear. The catheter is attached to an injection cap and glued in place. (*C*) It is then taped to a bandage to avoid slippage and to separate the injection port from the skin surface.

do not drink when allowed access to water. If electrolytes other than sodium and chloride are required, they should be added to the oral fluids. To the author's knowledge, there have not been any clinical studies to determine the efficacy of hypertonic saline in comparison with isotonic solutions.

The rumen is an incredibly useful reservoir into which one may administer large volumes of water and rehydration solutions, and should be used whenever possible. For conditions whereby the gastrointestinal tract is functional, there is no reason not to administer intraluminal fluids along with intravenous fluids. There are several effective delivery systems for rapid and efficient intraluminal administration of electrolyte solutions. There are also several commercially available electrolyte and supplement packages to formulate the solutions. The concentration of electrolytes in the solutions varies dramatically, and it should be emphasized that nonalkalinizing oral electrolyte solutions are indicated in adult ruminants. Products that contain bicarbonate or acetate are designed for calves with diarrhea that generally have a metabolic acidosis, and would not be appropriate for adult cattle in most cases. By simply adding NaCl (7 g/L), KCl (1.25 g/L), and $CaCl_2$ (0.5 g/L) to 1 L of water (or 140 g NaCl, 25 g KCl, and 10 g $CaCl_2$ in 20 L or roughly 5 gallons of water), a homemade nonalkalinizing oral electrolyte solution for adult ruminants can be created that will effectively rehydrate animals without alkalinizing blood pH. One should always carefully evaluate the contents of the solution before deciding to administer it. An extensive list of commercially available solutions that can be compounded has been published.[25]

REFERENCES

1. Roussel AJ, Cohen ND, Holland PS, et al. Alterations in acid-base balance and serum electrolyte concentrations in cattle: 632 cases (1984-1994). J Am Vet Med Assoc 1998;212:1769–75.
2. Schotman AJ. The acid-base balance in clinically healthy and diseased cattle. Neth J Vet Sci 1971;4(1):5–23.
3. Welker B. Practical and appropriate fluid therapy. Bovine Clinics 1985;5(2):6–8.
4. George JW, Hird DW, George LW. Serum biochemical abnormalities in goats with uroliths: 107 cases (1992-2003). J Am Vet Med Assoc 2007;230(1):101–5.
5. Simpson DF, Erb HN, Smith DF. Base excess as a prognostic and diagnostic indicator in cows with abomasal volvulus or right displacement of the abomasum. Am J Vet Res 1985;46(4):796–7.
6. Whitlock RH, Tennant BC, Tasker JB. Acid-base disturbances in cattle with left abomasal displacements: right abomasal displacement, abomasal torsion, vagal indigestion syndrome, and intestinal obstructions (intussusception and cecal volvulus). In: Proceedings of Third International Conference on Production Disease in Farm Animals. Wageningen; 1976. p. 67–9.
7. Gingerich DA, Murdick PW. Experimentally induced intestinal obstruction in sheep: paradoxical aciduria in metabolic alkalosis. Am J Vet Res 1975;36(5):663–8.
8. Oetzel GR. Oral calcium supplementation in peripartum dairy cows. Vet Clin North Am Food Anim Pract 2013;29:447–54.
9. Sockett DC, Knight AP, Fettman MJ, et al. Metabolic changes due to experimentally induced rupture of the bovine urinary bladder. Cornell Vet 1986;76:198–212.
10. Donecker JM, Bellamy JE. Blood chemical abnormalities in cattle with ruptured bladders and ruptured urethras. Can Vet J 1982;23:355–7.
11. Kasari TR, Naylor JM. Clinical evaluation of intravenous sodium bicarbonate, sodium L-lactate, and sodium acetate for the treatment of acidosis in diarrheic calves. J Am Vet Med Assoc 1985;187:392–7.

12. Naylor JM, Forsyth GW. The alkalinizing effects of metabolizable bases in the healthy calf. Can J Vet Res 1986;50:509–16.
13. Berchtold JF, Constable PD, Smith GW, et al. Effects of intravenous hyperosmotic sodium bicarbonate on arterial and cerebrospinal fluid acid-base status and cardiovascular function in calves with experimentally induced respiratory and strong ion acidosis. J Vet Intern Med 2005;19(2):240–51.
14. Constable PD, Walker PG, Morin DE, et al. Clinical and laboratory assessment of hydration status of neonatal calves with diarrhea. J Am Vet Med Assoc 1998;212: 991–6.
15. Repetto HA, Penna R. Apparent bicarbonate space in children. Scientific World Journal 2006;6:148–53.
16. Roussel AJ. Principles and mechanics of fluid therapy in calves. Compend Cont Educ Pract Vet 1983;5(6):S332–6.
17. Naylor JM. Clinical evaluation of sodium bicarbonate, sodium L-lactate, and sodium acetate for the treatment of acidosis in diarrheic calves. J Am Vet Med Assoc 1985;187(4):392–7.
18. Papadopoulos P, Raptopoulos D, Dessiris A, et al. Experimental intestinal obstruction in cattle. Part 2: Changes in blood, urine and rumen content chemistry. Zentralbl Veterinarmed A 1985;32:276–88.
19. Cornelius LM. Fluid therapy in small animal practice. J Am Vet Med Assoc 1980; 176(2):110–4.
20. Gruenberg W, Morin DE, Krackley JK, et al. Effect of rapid intravenous administration of 50% dextrose solution on phosphorus homeostasis in postparturient dairy cows. J Vet Intern Med 2006;20(6):1471–8.
21. Carlson GP. Energy loss in fluid therapy. N Engl J Med 1971;285:1328–9.
22. Koppinen J, Oijala M. Ambulatory rehydration: endotoxins in farm water. Acta Vet Scand 1987;28:253–4.
23. Corke MJ. Economical preparation of fluids for intravenous use in cattle practice. Vet Rec 1988;122:305–7.
24. Roussel AJ, Taliaoferro L, Navarre CB, et al. Catheterization of the auricular vein in cattle in cattle: 68 cases. J Am Vet Med Assoc 1996;208:905–7.
25. Constable PD. Fluid and electrolyte therapy in ruminants. Vet Clin Food Anim 2003;19:557–97.

Fluid Therapy in Small Ruminants and Camelids

Meredyth Jones, DVM, MS[a],*, Christine Navarre, DVM, MS[b]

KEYWORDS

- Fluid therapy • Sheep • Goat • Llama • Alpaca • Crystalloid • Colloid
- Parenteral nutrition

KEY POINTS

- Animals estimated to be more than 8% dehydrated should receive intravenous resuscitation at least initially, and then may be maintained on intravenous or oral fluid therapy.
- Hypoglycemia, hyperkalemia, and acidosis are the most life-threatening abnormalities, and require most immediate correction.
- Crystalloid solutions should be used cautiously in animals with hypoproteinemia because of the risk of pulmonary edema. Synthetic or natural colloid solutions are preferred in these patients.
- Hypertonic solutions are useful for short-term improvement of cardiac output, drawing water from the interstitium into the vasculature; they are contraindicated in hyperosmolar syndromes such as carbohydrate overload.
- Dextrose-containing solutions are indicated for use in hypoglycemic animals or those with hepatic lipidosis syndromes, but must be administered judiciously to achieve energy supplementation without inducing glucose diuresis. Insulin may be indicated to improve glucose utilization.
- Parenteral nutrition is indicated in patients with anorexia, those with severe systemic disease, and those with evidence of protein loss, and should be initiated early in the therapeutic period to achieve maximum efficacy.

INTRODUCTION

Body water, electrolytes, and acid-base balance are important considerations in the evaluation and treatment of animals with any disease process, with restoration of these a priority as adjunctive therapy. The goals of fluid therapy should be to maintain cardiac output and tissue perfusion, and to correct acid-base and electrolyte abnormalities.

The authors have no disclosures.
[a] Food Animal Field Services, Department of Large Animal Clinical Sciences, College of Veterinary Medicine, Texas A&M University, 4475 TAMU, College Station, TX 77843, USA; [b] LSU AgCenter, 105 Francioni Hall–LSU, Baton Rouge, LA 70803-4210, USA
* Corresponding author.
E-mail address: mjones@cvm.tamu.edu

PATIENT EVALUATION

A thorough physical examination is an important component of the evaluation of any patient, aiding in the diagnosis of the primary disease condition and the extent to which fluid and electrolyte therapy is indicated.

Hydration Deficit

Hydration deficit is best determined by reduction in body weight from the normally hydrated state, but this baseline body weight is infrequently available when the dehydrated patient is evaluated. Mental state, skin turgor, color and texture of mucous membrane, temperature of the extremities, and recession of the globe are all used in combination to estimate hydration status, but these criteria have not been validated in ruminants or camelids (**Table 1**). Alterations in packed cell volume (PCV) and total plasma protein (TPP) may also be used as indicators of hydration status, but are limited in their utility. The reference interval for PCV is fairly wide, making it an insensitive indicator of hydration, and baseline values for an individual are rarely available. Moreover, owing to the prevalence of diseases in sheep, goats, and camelids that alter PCV and TPP (internal parasitism, failure of passive transfer, chronic inflammatory disease), these values must be interpreted in light of the history and physical examination findings.

Electrolyte and Acid-Base Alterations

Serum biochemistry and blood gas analysis are the most appropriate tools for assessment of electrolyte, glucose, and acid-base abnormalities. Results of this testing may help prioritize fluid components for replacement. In general, hypoglycemia, hyperkalemia, and acidosis represent abnormalities that are most life-threatening and require the most immediate correction.

Fluid Administration

Route

The first decision to be made when initiating fluid therapy is whether fluids should be administered parenterally or enterally. In ruminants and camelids, large volumes of fluids may be administered into the rumen or first compartment, allowing for effective treatment of mild to moderate dehydration. In camelids specifically, the benefit of repeated oral fluid therapy should be weighed against the risks. Oral intubation is stressful in camelids and may induce cortisol-mediated lipolysis, particularly if repeated.[1] Therefore, the authors rarely use oral fluid therapy in camelids. In general, the animals most likely to benefit from oral fluid therapy are those that are mentally alert, have good gastrointestinal motility, and are less than 8% dehydrated. Animals

Table 1
Physical examination parameters for estimation of hydration deficit in ruminants and camelids

	Mild, 4%–6%	Moderate, 7%–9%	Severe, >10%
Cervical skin tent	4–5 s	5–7 s	>7 s
Globe recession	2–3 mm	3–4 mm	6–8 mm
Oral mucosa	Moist, warm, pink	Tacky, warm, pale	Dry, cool, pale
Extremities	Warm	Cool	Cold
Demeanor	Standing, bright	Sternal, slow	Lateral, depressed

Adapted from Constable PD, Walker PG, Morin DE, et al. Clinical and laboratory assessment of hydration status of neonatal calves with diarrhea. J Am Vet Med Assoc 1998;212:991–6; and Roussel AJ. Fluid therapy in mature cattle. Vet Clin N Am Food Anim Pract 1990;6(1):111–23.

not meeting these criteria are best managed with at least initial parenteral fluid resuscitation and correction of acid-base and electrolyte abnormalities.

In small ruminants, jugular catheterization is the most practical means of administering intravenous fluid therapy. In sheep and goats, over-the-needle catheters are typically used and placed with relative ease. In camelids, placement of jugular catheters can be more challenging and, although over-the-needle catheters are acceptable, peel-away catheters (**Fig. 1**) or J-wire catheters may result in easier and more reliable placement. A stab incision made with a #15 scalpel blade helps facilitate the placement of over-the-needle catheters in these species, particularly camelids. Recommended catheter sizes for jugular catheterization are summarized in **Table 2**.

Volume and rate

When determining appropriate fluid volume and rate to be administered, one must consider:

- Replacement of hydration deficit
- Maintenance fluid needs
- Replacement of ongoing losses
- Plasma protein concentration

Replacement of hydration deficit The volume required for hydration replacement is calculated using the following formula:

$$(\text{estimated \% dehydration}) \times (\text{body weight in kg}) = \text{liters of fluid needed to replace deficit}$$

As a general rule, hydration replacement should occur over approximately 4 hours, with maintenance and ongoing losses administered over the remaining hours in the day. In animals with low total protein and in camelids, hydration replacement may need to be slower, with half of the volume replaced in 4 to 6 hours and the remainder given over 12 to 24 hours.

Maintenance fluid requirement Maintenance fluid requirements account for normal water losses attributable to urination, defecation, respiration, sweat, and other

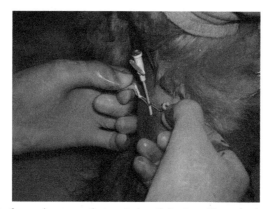

Fig. 1. Placement of a peel-away catheter. A sheath is placed into the jugular vein, as in an over-the-needle catheter setup, and the needle is removed. The long, soft catheter is fed into the sheath, which is then peeled into two halves and out of the vein, leaving the catheter in place.

Table 2
Recommended catheter sizes for jugular catheterization

Patient	Adult Sheep, Goat	Kid, Lamb	Adult Llama, Alpaca	Cria
Catheter size	16 gauge 3.25″ (8.3 cm)	18 gauge 2″ (5.1 cm)	14–16 gauge 3.25–5.5″ (8.3–14 cm)	16–18 gauge 2–3.5″ (5.1–8.9 cm)

evaporation, and differ based on physiologic status (lactation, pregnancy) and age. Neonates have higher total body water volume than adults, and require a higher maintenance fluid volume.

Maintenance fluid needs can be estimated using the following general guidelines:

- Adults: 50 mL/kg/24 hours or 1 mL/lb/h
- Neonates: 70 to 80 mL/kg/24 h or 2 mL/lb/h

These numbers are typically used in all species and are supported by established water requirements of goats, which range from 30 to 66.6 mL/kg/d with a mean of 44.8 mL/kg/d.[2] Neonates are typically assigned a higher maintenance volume, with 70 mL/kg found to be acceptable in calves.[3]

If fluid rates are difficult to control or are in animals likely to disrupt the fluid line, replacement fluids may be divided and administered every 3 hours by calculating the total volume needed for a 3-hour period and providing this as a single bolus. This approach is not appropriate with solutions that contain greater than 2% dextrose or with parenteral nutrition (PN) solutions.

Ongoing losses Ongoing losses include fluid, protein, and electrolytes, which are lost as a result of a continuing disease process, such as diarrhea or internal or external loss of fluid. Quantifying ongoing losses can be challenging and, in the absence of the ability to measure these directly, parameters such as PCV, TPP, serum electrolyte panel, and body weight may be used to monitor the success of fluid therapy to sustain body fluid, protein, and electrolyte balance.

FLUID TYPE

The 4 basic types of solutions used in clinical practice, which vary in composition, cost, and usefulness depending on the pathologic processes, are crystalloid solutions, colloid solutions, PN, and blood products. The article by Balcomb and Foster elsewhere in this issue addresses the use of whole blood and blood products. A summary algorithm to assist in fluid selection is provided in **Fig. 2**.

Crystalloid Solutions

Crystalloid solutions represent the most common fluids used in veterinary practice, and contain water, electrolytes (particularly sodium), and/or dextrose. Crystalloids may be classified as balanced, resembling the composition of the extracellular fluid, or unbalanced, designed to replace specific components.

Examples of crystalloid solutions used in veterinary practice include:

- Isotonic solutions
  - Balanced solutions
    - Polyionic solutions (Ringer's solutions; Normosol [Hospira, Lake Forest, IL]; Plasma-Lyte [Baxter, Deerfield, IL])
  - Unbalanced solutions
    - 0.9% NaCl solution

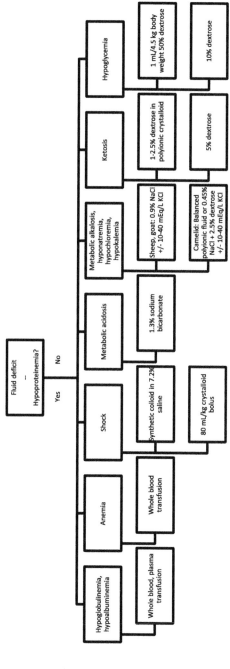

Fig. 2. Suggested fluid compositions for various clinical and metabolic conditions in small ruminants and camelids.

- 1.3% $NaHCO_3$ solution
- 5% dextrose solution

The isotonic crystalloids have an osmolality similar to that of plasma and equilibrate rapidly with the interstitial fluid. Only 20% to 25% of the infused volume of the administered solution remains in the intravascular space 1 hour after infusion. For this reason, crystalloids are well suited for rehydration of body tissues and restoration of electrolyte and acid-base abnormalities, but are not ideal for long-term maintenance of cardiac output. This characteristic of crystalloid solutions must also be considered when treating patients with hypoproteinemia, a common condition in small ruminants and camelids. Proteins serve to retain fluid within the vasculature, and the use of crystalloids in hypoproteinemic patients is associated with the development of edema and, of particular concern, pulmonary edema.

Hypertonic Solutions

Hypertonic solutions have a higher osmolality relative to plasma, the most common of which is hypertonic saline (7.2% NaCl), which has been used successfully in the resuscitation of sheep after hemorrhage.[4] These solutions are contraindicated in hyperosmolar conditions, which may occur in ill camelids and with camelids with grain overload. Hypertonic solutions are reviewed in the article by Smith and Berchtold elsewhere in this issue.

Hypotonic Solutions

Hypotonic solutions are rarely used in veterinary medicine. Although there are some specific conditions for which they have value, these are not common, and rapid administration of solutions that are hypotonic relative to a patient's serum can cause development of cerebral edema and lysis of brain cells.

Acidifying Solutions

Saline and Ringer's solution are acidifying solutions that are appropriate as a sole solution or as a base solution for animals presenting with metabolic alkalosis, as may occur with gastrointestinal obstruction or stasis and anorexia. Because of its high sodium content, saline is also useful for correcting hyponatremia, as occurs with obstructive urolithiasis and ruptured urinary bladder. Alkalotic ruminants are frequently anorexic, resulting in hypokalemia, and supplementation of these base solutions with 10 to 40 mEq/L of potassium chloride is frequently indicated.

Alkalinizing Solutions

Metabolic acidosis is encountered in patients with carbohydrate overload, diarrhea from enteritis, pregnancy toxemia, and a few other conditions. Isotonic sodium bicarbonate (1.3% $NaHCO_3$) and hypertonic sodium bicarbonate (5% or 8.4% $NaHCO_3$) may be used alone or be added to other solutions to directly correct metabolic acidosis. To determine the bicarbonate replacement needed for a patient, the following equations may be used:

Neonates: mEq bicarbonate needed = base deficit $\times$ body weight in kg $\times$ 0.6

Adults: mEq bicarbonate needed = base deficit $\times$ body weight in kg $\times$ 0.3

For these formulas, the base deficit may be directly obtained from a blood gas analysis, or estimated by subtracting the patient's serum total CO_2 (or plasma bicarbonate) from the normal serum total CO_2 value of 24 mEq/mL. The constants 0.6 and 0.3 represent the approximate proportion of extracellular fluid volume relative to total body weight, which is different for neonates compared with mature animals. From this formula, the total milliequivalents of bicarbonate needed to completely correct the acidosis can be calculated. Intravenous administration of 1.3% $NaHCO_3$ is frequently used for this replacement, and contains approximately 156 mEq bicarbonate/L. The hypertonic 5.0% $NaHCO_3$ contains 0.6 mEq/mL of sodium bicarbonate, whereas 8.4% $NaHCO_3$ contains 1 mEq/mL. Isotonic 1.3% $NaHCO_3$ solution may be formulated by beginning with 260 mL of 5% $NaHCO_3$ or 156 mL of 8.4% $NaHCO_3$ and adding a sufficient quantity of sterile water to make 1 L. Hypertonic $NaHCO_3$ solutions should be used with caution until proved to be safe for camelids. Recently, hypertonic $NaHCO_3$ solutions have been shown to be effective in treating D-lactate acidosis in calves.[5]

In some cases, such as neonatal diarrhea and severe grain overload, the entire calculated deficit of bicarbonate may need to be administered to correct the acidosis, but in most cases partial correction by administration of about half of the deficit over 2 to 4 hours will be followed by complete correction, after fluid resuscitation allows the normal physiologic compensatory mechanisms to function in the treated animal.

Solutions including lactated Ringer's, Normosol-R (Hospira), and Plasma-Lyte A (Baxter) are also considered alkalinizing fluids, owing to the presence of the metabolizable bases lactate, acetate, or gluconate. These bases are metabolized by various tissues, depending on the metabolizable base, resulting in a net increase in the strong ion difference that corrects the metabolic acidosis. However, the alkalinizing effect will be delayed relative to the administration of $NaHCO_3$ solution, owing to the time required for metabolism. When using a product containing lactate, it is important to remember that only the L-lactate isomer is metabolized to bicarbonate even though the solution contains equal parts of the D- and L-isomers. When perfusion of the liver is altered, the D-isomer will not be metabolized efficiently and may exacerbate lactic acidosis. Combined with the delayed alkalization potential of the metabolizable bases relative to bicarbonate, this makes these solutions less desirable for resuscitation of a moderate to severe metabolic acidosis.

A D-lactic acidosis syndrome of lambs has been described, resulting in severe metabolic acidosis[6] believed to result from increased substrate presentation to the large intestine. A similar syndrome has been described in goat kids.[7] These syndromes have been successfully corrected through the oral administration of 50 mmol HCO_3 administered as 50 mL 8.4% $NaHCO_3$ solution,[8] or intravenous administration of 5% sodium bicarbonate, along with oral supplementation, based on measured base deficit.[7]

Dextrose Solutions

Dextrose-containing solutions without electrolytes have a relatively narrow spectrum of utility because of the rapid metabolism of the dextrose component, leaving free water to dilute other blood components. These solutions are useful in the treatment of hypoglycemia in neonates, particularly if hypothermic, and in animals with pregnancy toxemia. Fifty percent dextrose is commercially available and may be administered undiluted at 1 mL/10 lb (4.5 kg) body weight during hypoglycemic crisis, or added to sterile water to make 10% dextrose (200 mL/L) and 5% isotonic dextrose (100 mL/L), which may be used alone or in combination with other fluids. Fifty percent dextrose may also be added to polyionic solutions to make 1% to 2.5% solutions (20–50 mL/L) to provide a source of energy.

Pregnancy toxemia is a common indication for the use of dextrose-containing solutions over a period of time. In sheep and goats, a variety of metabolic derangements have been documented as part of the pregnancy toxemia, including hyperketonemia, ketonuria, metabolic acidosis, hypocalcemia, hypoglycemia, and decreased liver function from hepatic lipidosis.[9] Hypoglycemia is an inconsistent finding in cases of pregnancy toxemia, and a finding of euglycemia or hyperglycemia should not dissuade one from considering pregnancy toxemia as a differential diagnosis.

Oral fluid therapy may be used to prevent the progression of very early pregnancy toxemia, and is frequently initiated by producers at the farm. In cases where the animal is recumbent or prefers to be recumbent, oral therapy should not be expected to halt or reverse the progression of pregnancy toxemia. Intravenous therapy is nearly always indicated in these cases, and should not be postponed.

Polyionic, balanced solutions containing dextrose are typically used as the basis for therapy for pregnancy toxemia; however, additional components such as calcium gluconate 23% (20–50 mL/L), $NaHCO_3$ (calculated from base deficit), and potassium (20–40 mEq/L) may be added to the base solution. Solutions should not be formulated to contain both calcium and bicarbonate ions because these 2 ions may form an insoluble precipitate. Glucose is usually provided to small ruminants and camelids as 2.5% dextrose in a polyionic solution or 5% dextrose in polyionic solution or water. The rate and concentration of dextrose should be adjusted in response to changes in the concentrations of glucose and ketones in the urine. The goal is to provide enough energy to reduce or eliminate ketone production yet not exceed the renal threshold for glucose, which will result in diuresis. Although the goal of negative results for both urine glucose and ketones is seldom achieved, monitoring urinary ketones and glucose is a sensitive and inexpensive method by which to evaluate the success of energy supplementation in these cases.

A major goal of therapy is to reestablish the appetite of the patient. Dextrose-containing fluids are not a replacement for enteral nutrition, as 5% dextrose given at maintenance rate provides only 25% of maintenance energy requirement while meeting none of the protein or other nutritional requirements of a late-gestation animal. At least partial PN (PPN) is indicated for many animals with pregnancy toxemia. Prolonged or repeated administration of dextrose-containing solutions may be associated with hypophosphatemia and subsequent recumbency, especially in anorexic animals.[10]

Dextrose-containing solutions should be used with caution in camelid species. Camelids have been shown to produce less insulin and to have decreased insulin sensitivity in comparison with other species.[11] When dextrose-containing fluids are used, the dextrose concentration should be low (usually 2.5% or lower) and blood glucose should be monitored, and exogenous insulin administration may be required during therapy. An exception to this is animals that are anorexic or experiencing hepatic lipidosis. In these cases, dextrose therapy and PN are indicated to reduce the progression of lipolysis, which leads to further depression of appetite and worsening of the condition. Insulin therapy is indicated for blood glucose concentrations exceeding 350 to 400 mg/dL, and the following doses are provided as starting points for subcutaneous therapy: regular insulin 0.25 U/kg, Ultralente 0.2 to 0.4 U/kg, Lente 0.25 to 0.5 U/kg.

A hyperosmolar syndrome has been described in ill neonatal camelids,[12,13] characterized by hyperglycemia, hypernatremia, and hyperosmolarity, which manifests as a fine head tremor, ataxia, and base-wide stance. Insulin resistance and glucose diuresis are believed to be among the contributors to this syndrome; therefore, solutions containing high concentrations of sodium and dextrose are typically avoided in neonatal camelids. Insulin therapy is indicated for this syndrome, with constant-rate regular insulin infusion advocated at an initial rate 0.02 U/kg/h.[13]

Colloidal Solutions

Colloidal solutions contain high molecular weight compounds that are retained in the intravascular space and serve to maintain or increase intravascular volume in animals with hypoproteinemia. These molecules act similarly to albumin by maintaining osmotic pressure within the vascular system. In fact, on a weight to weight basis, 6% dextran 70 is actually 2.5 times more osmotically active than albumin.[4]

Colloidal solutions may be divided into natural and synthetic compounds.

- Natural colloid solutions
  - Whole blood
  - Plasma
- Synthetic colloid solutions
  - Hetastarch
  - Dextrans
  - Modified gelatin solutions

Despite their higher cost, colloids are more appropriate than crystalloids for use in hypoproteinemic patients and those requiring longer-term stabilization of cardiac output. In one study of induced hemorrhage and resuscitation in sheep, the addition of 6% dextran 70 to 7.2% NaCl resulted in maintenance of a significantly higher cardiac output in comparison with other hypertonic solutions by redistribution of interstitial fluid into the vasculature.[4]

The use of hetastarch has been evaluated in healthy llamas.[14] Administration of 50 mL/kg hetastarch over 60 minutes to healthy llamas resulted in hemodilution, as indicated by significant decreases in hematocrit, hemoglobin, total serum protein, and albumin concentrations, indicating the ability of hetastarch to expand plasma volume. These effects were greater than those observed after administration of lactated Ringer's solution. Hetastarch also significantly increased plasma colloid osmotic pressure for 96 hours after infusion.

Orally Administered Solutions

Oral fluid therapy represents an economical and effective means for replacing mild to moderate fluid and electrolyte deficits. In addition, oral therapy is indicated in cases of severe hypokalemia and hypophosphatemia, where intravenous administration carries a greater risk for complications and is frequently less effective than oral therapy.

To achieve effective absorption of water, oral fluids must contain sufficient sodium to facilitate transport across the intestinal mucosa. Ideally oral solutions should contain at least 90 mmol/L of sodium. Ruminants with anorexia and gastrointestinal stasis frequently have low concentrations of plasma potassium and chloride, making it important that oral replacement solutions contain extraphysiologic concentrations of these electrolytes.

- Oral electrolyte solution for adult ruminants (per liter of water)
  - 7 g NaCl
  - 1.5 g KCl
  - 1 g CaCl$_2$

Table 3 lists common conversions for salts used in oral fluids.

Severe hypophosphatemia may be encountered in animals with prolonged anorexia or parasitism. Phosphate is the bioactive form of phosphorus, making phosphite salt forms found in commercially available intravenous solutions inadequate for

Table 3
Conversion of grams of listed feed-grade salt per teaspoon (g/t)

Salt	g/t
NaCl	6.1
KCl	6
NaHCO$_3$	5
CaCl$_2$	4

phosphorus replacement. Phosphate salts may be found in commercially available phosphate enemas, but must be carefully diluted for intravenous use, and intravenous administration is associated with an inadequate duration of the increase in serum phosphorus in cattle.[15] Oral supplementation of phosphorus is preferable and, in alpacas, the administration of 1 to 2 (4.5 oz/13 mL each) monobasic/dibasic sodium phosphate enemas in oral fluids by one of the authors (M.J.) has resulted in increases in serum phosphorus level of 2 to 3 mg/dL.

PARENTERAL NUTRITION

PN is an effective means for providing nutrients to anorectic or hypophagic animals that warrant aggressive therapy. PN can be costly, requires careful monitoring, and should be initiated early in the course of treatment to maximize its efficacy. Indications for PN include anorexia for longer than 3 days, severe systemic disease, and evidence of protein loss. Total PN (TPN) is designed to meet all of an animal's nutritional needs, with base components of dextrose, amino acids, and lipids. PPN is limited in either the components it provides or the amount of components relative to the animal's needs. The cost of TPN precludes its use in many cases, but PPN formulations exist to provide valuable nutrients for maintenance and repair at a reasonable cost. The lipid component is the most costly, and is typically the component omitted when formulating PPN.

A retrospective study was performed evaluating PN in alpacas suffering from gastrointestinal disease, liver disease, neoplasia, and other conditions.[16] Twenty of 22 animals had severe metabolic derangements before therapy, and at least 1 complication from PN occurred in 21 of 22 animals, including hyperglycemia, lipemia, hypokalemia, and refeeding syndrome. Overall survival rate to discharge was 45% and was unrelated to diagnosis, although the study population was small.

- PPN solution for sheep and goats
  - 5 L commercial balanced electrolyte solution
  - 500 mL 50% dextrose
  - 1 L 8.5% amino acids (commercially available preparation)
  - 20 mL B-complex vitamins
  - Potassium chloride (20–40 mEq/L) and calcium gluconate 23% (20–50 mL/L) as indicated
  This solution has been used by one of the authors (C.N.) in adult sheep, goats, and camelids. It is administered at a rate of 5% of body weight per day, and may be administered without the use of a fluid pump.
- PPN for camelids
  - Clore and colleagues,[16] 2011
    - Amino acid to provide 4 to 6 g/100 kcal protein
    - 50% dextrose to provide 40% to 60% of nonprotein calories
    - 20% lipid to provide remaining 40% to 60% of nonprotein calories

- Additional B vitamins with or without trace minerals
- OR
- Commercial dextrose/amino acid solution to provide 4.25 g/100 kcal protein plus 100% nonprotein calories from dextrose
- Calcium gluconate, trace minerals, magnesium sulfate, and B complex added as indicated by intake and serum biochemistry

  These protocols were compounded and used at 2 academic institutions for a variety of disease conditions in alpacas along with other specific and supportive therapies.
  - Van Saun and colleagues,[1] 2000
    - 880 mL of 50% dextrose
    - 2000 mL of 8.5% amino acids
    - 100 mL of 23% calcium gluconate
    - 5 mL vitamin B complex
    - 30 mL potassium chloride (4 mEq/mL)
    - Sufficient quantity to 4 L in a base solution of lactated Ringer's solution
    - Administered at a rate of 2.5 mL/kg/h
    - 30 U NPH insulin (animal weighed 102 kg) was administered subcutaneously every 12 hours initially and then whenever blood glucose exceeded 400 mg/dL

      This protocol was used in an adult female llama with hepatic lipidosis for

---

Box 1
General guidelines for administration of parenteral nutrition (PN)

Initiation

The components should be mixed aseptically, with amino acids added first, followed by any lipid component, then dextrose

A large-gauge, long catheter is preferable and must be aseptically placed

A separate catheter should be placed if other drugs are to be administered, or the PN catheter should be flushed well before and after drug administration

When PN is initiated, it should be at 25% to 50% of target rate for a few hours. If hyperglycemia does not develop, the rate is increased to the target rate, usually 5% of body weight daily

Daily

The catheter should be examined 3 to 4 times per day for evidence of phlebitis or other complications

Vital parameters should be monitored every 8 hours

Blood glucose may need to be monitored every 6 to 8 hours

The PN solution and all lines should be changed daily

Body weight should be monitored daily

Assessment of packed cell volume and total plasma protein should be performed daily, and the plasma evaluated visually for evidence of lipemia

Assessment of serum electrolytes, creatinine, and liver enzymes should be performed daily, in addition to urinalysis

Cessation

If insulin is administered with PN, insulin therapy should be stopped 24 hours before cessation of PN

When PN is discontinued, it should be decreased slowly over 24 to 48 hours

1 week, and PN was gradually discontinued over 3 days once the clinical condition had stabilized and the animal was eating.

The metabolism of carbohydrates and lipids by camelids is complex and complicated.[11,17] Therefore, PN solutions for camelids are sometimes formulated with a higher ratio of amino acids to nonprotein sources of energy in comparison with PN solutions for other species. Close monitoring for hyperlipemia and the need for insulin administration is critical. General guidelines for administration of PN are shown in **Box 1**.

Refeeding syndrome, an important potential complication in the initial days of recovery from starvation or treatment with PN,[16,18] is characterized by hypophosphatemia, hypokalemia, hypomagnesemia, and other electrolyte and metabolic abnormalities, with severe effects on most body systems. Patients at risk for refeeding syndrome should undergo gradual refeeding or PN administration, be monitored closely for its development, and be supplemented with target electrolytes and minerals.

REFERENCES

1. Van Saun RJ, Callihan BR, Tornquist SJ. Nutritional support for treatment of hepatic lipidosis in a llama. J Am Vet Med Assoc 2000;217(10):1531–5.
2. Nutrient requirements of small ruminants: sheep, goats, cervids, and New World camelids. Washington, DC: The National Academies Press; 2007.
3. Gottardo F, Mattiello S, Cozzi G, et al. The provision of drinking water to veal calves for welfare purposes. J Anim Sci 2002;80(9):2362–72.
4. Smith J, Kramer GC, Perron P, et al. A comparison of several hypertonic solutions for resuscitation in bled sheep. J Surg Res 1985;39:517–28.
5. Lorenz I, Vogt S. Investigations on the association of D-lactate blood concentrations with the outcome of therapy of acidosis, and with posture and demeanour in young calves with diarrhoea. J Vet Med A Physiol Pathol Clin Med 2006;53(9):490–4.
6. Angell JW, Jones G, Grove-White DH, et al. A prospective on farm cohort study investigating the epidemiology and pathophysiology of drunken lamb syndrome. Vet Rec 2013;172:154–7.
7. Bleul U, Schwantag S, Stocker H, et al. Floppy kid syndrome caused by D-lactic acidosis in goat kids. J Vet Intern Med 2006;20:1003–8.
8. Angell JW, Jones GL, Voight K, et al. Successful correction of D-lactic acid neurotoxicity (drunken lamb syndrome) by bolus administration of oral sodium bicarbonate. Vet Rec 2013;173:193–5.
9. Van Saun RJ. Pregnancy toxemia in a flock of sheep. J Am Vet Med Assoc 2000;217(10):1536–9.
10. Grunberg W, Morin DE, Drackley JK, et al. Effect of continuous intravenous administration of a 50% dextrose solution on phosphorus homeostasis in dairy cows. J Am Vet Med Assoc 2006;229:413–20.
11. Firshman AM, Cebra CK, Schanbacher BJ, et al. Evaluation of insulin secretion and action in New World camelids. Am J Vet Res 2013;74:96–101.
12. Cebra CK. Hyperglycemia, hypernatremia and hyperosmolarity in 6 neonatal llamas and alpacas. J Am Vet Med Assoc 2000;217(11):1701–4.
13. Buchheit TM, Sommardahl CS, Frank N, et al. Use of a constant rate infusion of insulin for the treatment of hyperglycemic, hypernatremic, hyperosmolar syndrome in an alpaca cria. J Am Vet Med Assoc 2010;236:562–6.
14. Carney KR, McKenzie EC, Mosley CA, et al. Evaluation of the effect of hetastarch and lactated Ringer's solution on plasma colloid osmotic pressure in healthy llamas. J Am Vet Med Assoc 2011;238:768–72.

15. Cheng YH, Goff JP, Horst RL. Restoring normal blood phosphorus concentrations in hypophosphatemic cattle with sodium phosphate. Vet Med 1998;93:240–3.
16. Clore ER, Freeman LM, Bedenice D, et al. Retrospective evaluation of parenteral nutrition in alpacas: 22 cases (2002-2008). J Vet Intern Med 2011;25:598–604.
17. Waitt LH, Cebra CK. Characterization of hypertriglyceridemia and response to treatment with insulin in llamas and alpacas: 31 cases (1995-2005). J Am Vet Med Assoc 2008;232:1362–7.
18. Marinella MA. The refeeding syndrome and hypophosphatemia. Nutr Rev 2003; 61(9):320–3.

Update on the Use of Blood and Blood Products in Ruminants

Christie Balcomb, BVSc[a],*, Derek Foster, DVM, PhD[b]

KEYWORDS

- Transfusion • Anemia • Hemolysis • Hypoproteinemia • Blood • Plasma

KEY POINTS

- A packed cell volume of less than 12% with clinical signs of a significant anemia or blood loss is an indication for a blood transfusion.
- Ten to 15 mL/kg of whole blood can be collected from a healthy donor animal at one time.
- Blood or plasma should be administered at a rate of 1 to 5 mL/kg/h initially and increased to 10 to 20 mL/kg/h.
- Neonatal ruminants with failure of passive transfer of immunity require 20 to 40 mL/kg of plasma to raise serum IgG sufficiently.

INTRODUCTION

The use of whole blood and/or blood products is occasionally indicated in ruminant practice. The primary goal of this article is to summarize previously published data relating to blood groups in ruminants and camelids, as well as blood collection and transfusion techniques applicable to both small ruminants and cattle.

Whole blood transfusions are required in conditions of hemorrhage or erythrolysis (intravascular or extravascular) because of a variety of causes, such as acute traumatic hemorrhage, parasitism, toxicosis, or immune-mediated anemia. Clinical signs of anemia include tachycardia, tachypnea, lethargy, weakness, respiratory distress, pale or discolored mucous membranes, and prolonged capillary refill time. Hematologic parameters consistent with anemia include a packed cell volume (PCV) of less than 20% and abnormal erythrocyte morphology, such as anisocytosis, reticulocytosis, or Heinz body formation. Serum biochemistry changes in anemic patients include

The authors have nothing to disclose.
[a] William R. Pritchard Veterinary Medical Teaching Hospital, University of California, 1 Shields Avenue, Davis, CA 95616, USA; [b] Department of Population Health and Pathobiology, College of Veterinary Medicine, North Carolina State University, 1060 William Moore Drive, Raleigh, NC 27607, USA
* Corresponding author.
E-mail address: cbalcomb@ucdavis.edu

prerenal or renal azotemia (elevated serum urea nitrogen or creatinine), elevated lactate, decreased oxygen saturation, and elevated potassium. Changes in the hemogram and serum chemistry depend largely on the severity of anemia, cause, and chronicity of disease.

Plasma transfusions can be warranted in cases of failure of passive transfer (FPT) of immunity in neonatal ruminants, in hypoproteinemia such as a protein-losing enteropathy, or in cases of specific clotting factor, platelet, or leukocyte disorders. Blood component transfusions of packed red blood cells (pRBCs) or platelet-rich plasma (PRP) are less frequently performed but can be indicated in certain situations.

NORMAL HEMATOLOGIC VALUES FOR RUMINANTS

There are broad reference ranges for ruminants, with significant breed differences in hematological values. Hematological differences may also reflect species, age, gender, and physiologic state (**Fig. 1**).[1] For the most part, these details are beyond the scope of this article; however, there are some features of ruminant hematology that are important to note when performing in-house hematology or in an emergency situation. Camelid erythrocytes are ellipsoid; therefore, commercial blood analyzers may misinterpret erythrocytes as platelets and give falsely low values.[2] Erythrocytes of most sheep and goat breeds are small and disc-shaped, and normal animals may have some variation in cell shape, with Angora goats having fusiform-shaped erythrocytes.[1]

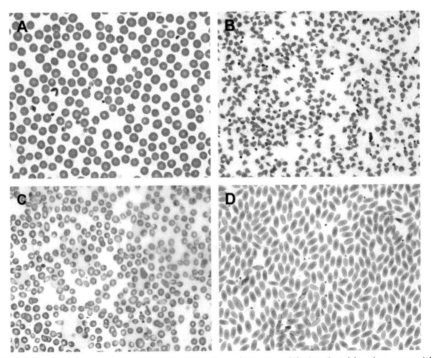

Fig. 1. (*A*) Bovine blood smear with normal erythrocytes. (*B*) Caprine blood smear with normal erythrocytes. Note anisocytosis and fusiform erythrocytes. (*C*) Ovine blood smear with normal erythrocytes. (*D*) Llama blood smear with normal erythrocytes. All images were taken at ×100 with Wright-Geimsa stain. (*Courtesy of* Kyle L. Webb, DVM, College of Veterinary Medicine, North Carolina State University.)

WHOLE BLOOD
Indications

The purpose of the circulating blood volume is to maintain adequate tissue oxygenation, provide nutrients and removal of waste products, and provide coagulation factors for hemostasis. Whole blood transfusions can be used to increase or maintain tissue oxygenation and to replace circulating blood volume. Cardiogenic shock occurs when 30% of the circulating blood volume is lost acutely. However, with more insidious blood loss, such as with chronic parasitism, animals can cope with extremely low PCVs of 8% to 10% before showing adverse clinical signs because there is adequate time for compensatory mechanisms to mitigate the effects of the anemia.

In general, whole blood transfusions are recommended when the PCV decreases to less than 15% to 20% in cases of acute blood loss or less than 10% to 15% in cases of chronic anemia.[3] A PCV of 12% or less following an acute episode of anemia is considered "critical" (**Table 1**). Other parameters to quantify the level of anemia include plasma proteins, clinical signs (pale mucous membranes, weakness, lethargy, tachycardia, tachypnea), hemoglobin concentration, and mixed venous oxygen partial pressure.[3] With handheld blood gas analyzers present in more veterinary practices, it is now possible to rapidly determine some of these parameters on the farm. Handheld blood gas analyzers can be useful in a field setting when there is no access to a centrifuge to determine PCV. One can multiply the hemoglobin concentrations (g/dL) by 3 to estimate PCV (%). Myocardial oxygenation is compromised at hemoglobin levels less than 5 g/dL (PCV 15%), increasing the risk of tissue hypoxia.[4] In human medicine, a "transfusion trigger" is often used, corresponding to hemoglobin levels of 7 to 9 g/dL.[5,6] The decision to transfuse whole blood should be based on a combination of history, clinical presentation, and clinicopathological data.

Table 1 Important quantities to remember	
Whole blood	
Critical anemia (PCV)	12%
Circulating blood volume (CBV)	8% of body weight (kg)
Donor collection volume	10–15 mL/kg or 20% of CBV
Initial administration rate	1–5 mL/kg/h for first 10–20 min
Rate of administration	10–20 mL/kg/h
Plasma	
Total protein indicating FPT	<5.2 g/dL (IgG<1000 mg/dL)
Volume required for FPT	20–40 mL/kg
Rate of administration	As above for whole blood transfusion
pRBC	
Volume required	Use donor PCV calculation
Platelet-rich plasma	
1 unit	Volume from 500 mL whole blood
Volume required	1 unit/10 kg body weight
Emergency drugs	
Flunixin meglumine (pre-med)	1.1 mg/kg intravenously
Epinephrine	0.002–0.003 mg/kg (intravenously), 0.01–0.02 mg/kg (intramuscularly)

Contraindications

Contraindications for whole blood transfusion are dictated by prognosis and a likely response to treatment, which is influenced by the underlying disease process. Acute, moderate to severe hemorrhage may respond well to transfusion therapy, whereas a chronic hemolytic anemia with on-going erythrocyte destruction may have a poor chance of success and may even require subsequent transfusions. Although rare in ruminants and camelids, there is a risk of transfusion reactions primarily due to issues such as volume overload and anaphylactic reactions in response to foreign antigens. These risks are discussed in detail later in the article. Owners of animals with a history of previous transfusions or anaphylactic reactions should be warned of the risks and potential for complications. Severely anemic cattle may experience a hypoxemic hyperexcitement, which may be dangerous for both patient and clinician.

Duration of Benefit

Whole blood transfusions provide the short-term benefit of replacing circulating blood volume and improving tissue oxygenation. However, these benefits begin to wane after a few days and subsequent transfusions may be necessary, especially in cases of nonregenerative anemia. There is some variation reported in the survival of red cells after transfusion based on species and method of labeling technique. Seventy-five percent of transfused red blood cells (RBCs) should still be in circulation at 24 hours after transfusion[7]; however, it is known that transfused erythrocytes have a reduced lifespan in circulation. Allogenic transfused erythrocytes have a half-life of about 5 days, and autologous transfused erythrocytes have a half-life of about 11 days in foals.[8] More recent research using biotinylation technique in horses indicated a half-life of allogenic RBCs of 20 days, which is longer than has been previously reported with radioactive labeling, but shorter than many other species.[9] The development of alloantibodies to donor RBC antigens occurs around 4 days after transfusion, resulting in removal of transfused erythrocytes and sensitization against this particular donor.[10] Additional transfusions may be required, but this comes at an increased risk of transfusion reactions and accelerated immune-modulated donor cell destruction. Daily PCV and total solids should be measured to monitor the potential for excessive loss or destruction of transfused erythrocytes.

Quantity Required

Traditionally, hemorrhagic shock occurs when blood loss exceeds 30% of total blood volume. Ideally, if a transfusion is required for hemorrhagic shock, at least half the estimated blood loss should be replaced, but some is better than none.[3] Total blood volume is estimated to be 8% of total body weight in kilograms. For example, a 50-kg calf has approximately 4 L total blood volume and would experience hemorrhagic shock with a loss of 1.2 L blood. At least half the volume lost (600 mL) of whole blood would be required for transfusion.

In cases of more chronic blood loss, a mathematical formula based on PCV may be appropriate and can be extrapolated from other species[4]:

$$\text{Blood volume to be infused (L)} = \frac{\text{Desired PCV}\,(\%) - \text{Recipient PCV}\,(\%)}{\text{Donor PCV}\,(\%)}$$

$$\times \text{ Recipient body weight (kg)} \times 0.08$$

Goats are considered to have a large capacity of splenic erythrocyte storage and can therefore accommodate a blood loss of 25% to 50% over a 24-h period.[11] In cases of chronic blood loss from parasitism, the PCV can be less than 10% without overt clinical signs of anemia unless the animal is stressed, is physically exerted, or has concurrent disease. In these cases, if oxygen demands can be kept minimal, replacement of intravascular fluid and/or protein may have priority over erythrocyte supplementation.

Donor Selection

The major concerns when selecting a blood donor are to minimize the risks of transfusion reactions and transmissible diseases to the recipient. Because of the numerous blood types in ruminants and camelids, the risk of reactions from a single transfusion is low. Donors should preferably have good temperament to facilitate collection. If necessary, sedation with xylazine (0.05-0.10 mg/kg intramuscularly) can be used to reduce stress and aid in catheter placement and collection.[12,13]

Blood groups/types
From the 1940s to the 1970s, there was a significant amount of research done on blood groups of domestic mammals. Scientists such as Rasmusen and Stormont elucidated the numerous blood group systems in ruminant species as well as the complicated blood type factors or phenogroups within these systems.[14–16] Little further study has been done since. Hemolytic tests via complement are the preferred method of blood typing in cattle, sheep, goats, and camelids because erythrocytes are not prone to agglutination, as they are in horses, cats, and dogs.[1] Because of the high variability of blood types and factors, especially for cattle, it is somewhat impractical for individual blood typing or factor identification to be performed before a transfusion. Determination of genetic blood group system or blood phenogroup may be more of academic interest and can be used to trace parentage, but is beyond the scope of this article.[17] Generally, single, unmatched, whole blood transfusions in food animals will be unlikely to result in a reaction; however, caution should be taken in any subsequent transfusions.

The previous version of this article[3] listed several commercial laboratories that performed ruminant blood typing, but as of 2013, those laboratories no longer offer commercial blood typing services. Most universities and blood banks generally do not type their donor animals and tend to only perform single transfusions, but can provide cross-matching for higher risk transfusions.

- Cattle: There are 11 genetic systems of blood groups (A, B, C, F, J, L, M, S, Z, R', T') with greater than 70 blood group factors recognized.[15,18] The J-factor is a glycolipid antigen primarily dissolved in plasma, not constitutively expressed on erythrocyte membranes, and only attaches to blood cells when sufficiently high concentrations are present. It is serologically related to the sheep R, pig A, and human A factors. It is possible for J-negative recipient to have J antibodies and thus have a reaction to the first transfusion of J-positive donor cells.[16]
- Sheep: Eight blood group systems (A, B, C, D, M, R, X) have been described with at least 22 blood group factors.[14,18] The R-factor, similar to the J-factor in cattle, is adsorbed onto erythrocyte membranes from plasma.
- Goats: There are at least 6 blood group systems (A, B, C, E, F, R) identified in goats, although much less developed than other species. Several goat blood group factors can cross-react with sheep blood-typing reagents.[18]
- Alpacas and llamas: There is not much study of blood group variation in camelids. Six blood group systems have been identified (A, B, C, D, E, F).[18]

Biosecurity and disease transmission
General husbandry and management practices that may increase the probability of sensitization to a different blood group involve vaccination, drug administration, or

blood collection without changing needles between individuals. Environmental factors such as ticks or biting flies may also be able to transmit erythrocytes between individuals.

An ideal bovine donor should be a healthy adult, nonpregnant, J-factor-negative, tested free of viral disease (bovine leukosis virus and bovine viral diarrhea virus), bacterial disease (brucellosis, tuberculosis, paratuberculosis), and erythroparasites (anaplasmosis and other rickettsial organisms indigenous to specific geographic regions). Donors should also be free from internal and external parasites, with no history of vaccination for anaplasmosis, Johne's disease, or brucellosis as an adult.[3] Ovine or caprine donors should be healthy adults, nonpregnant, and free of diseases, such as caprine arthritis encephalitis virus, brucellosis, tuberculosis, Q fever (*Coxiella burnetti*), *Sarcocystis ovicanis, Corynebacterium pseudotuberculosis, Anaplasma ovis,* and *Mycoplasma ovis comb. nov.* (formerly *Eperythrozoon ovis*). Camelids, similarly, should be healthy without disease, including *Mycoplasma haemolamae*. It is important to note that blood products from llamas can be safely given to alpacas, and vice versa. Donors should have a PCV and serum protein within the normal reference range for species. If blood or blood products cannot be obtained from a known disease-free source, the next best candidate would be an individual from within the same herd. As noted above, the animal should be healthy, ideally free from parasitism, and with a normal PCV and serum protein concentration.

Since publication of the previous edition of this article,[3] there has been significant research into the transmission of transmissible spongiform encephalopathies (TSE) through blood and blood product transfusion in sheep, as a model to determine the risk of TSE transmission via blood transfusions in humans.[19–26] TSEs are infective neurodegenerative diseases that affect many species including variant Cruetzfeldt-Jakob disease in humans, scrapie in sheep and goats, bovine spongiform encephalopathy in cattle, and chronic wasting disease in deer and elk. This disease is characterized by the mutation of the PrP^C prion to the infective PrP^{Sc} isoform. Expression of this protein is found in the brain and lymphoreticular tissues. However, this protein mutation can be expressed on peripheral blood mononuclear cells, which can be detected with protein misfolded cyclic amplification or a ligand-based immunoassay. The latter assay is less sensitive, but has a shorter turnaround time.[27] Whole blood or buffy coat transfusions from experimentally infected sheep with naturally occurring scrapie infections given to susceptible, scrapie-free sheep resulted in development of clinical disease.[19–23,25,26] Transfusion of any blood component (whole blood, plasma, pRBCs, platelets, and buffy coat) is capable of transmitting TSE to susceptible sheep, and leukoreduction techniques described for use in human transfusion medicine are ineffective at eliminating the risk of disease transmission.[23] As little as 0.2 mL whole blood transfused from asymptomatic donors is sufficient to transmit scrapie to 100% of recipients.[26]

The National Scrapie Eradication Program was started in 2003, and the most current report states that 0.0151% of cull sheep were positive for scrapie at slaughter, representing a 90% reduction in prevalence over the past decade.[28] Although the prevalence of the disease is low, newly positive flocks and herds of goats are still being identified. Therefore, there is still risk of transmission through blood products used for transfusions from subclinically infected animals.

Autotransfusion

Autotransfusion (autologous transfusion) involves transfusion of the recipient's own blood, either collected before expected hemorrhage or from a body cavity after trauma or intraoperative or postoperative hemorrhage.[29,30] Advantages of autotransfusion include decreased risk of infectious disease transmission and transfusion reactions. This technique can be used in ruminant species if an appropriate donor is not available and as long as blood is collected aseptically and is free from bacterial or neoplastic cell contamination. Transfusion of blood obtained from body cavities may require additional blood filters to remove microemboli (replace filters with every 2 L of blood), but it needs less anticoagulant because of inactivation of many clotting factors.[4] There are still complications with this type of transfusion technique, such as hemolysis, microembolization, and potential spread of infectious agents or neoplastic cells.

Collection Technique

Techniques for blood collection of cattle have been described previously[3,4,12,13] but are summarized here. Up to 20% of a donor's total blood volume (10–15 mL/kg of body weight) can be harvested at one time.[3,31,32] Normal total blood volume in ruminant species is estimated at 8% of body weight (eg, a 500-kg cow has approximately 40 L blood, so 8 L can be safely harvested; see **Table 2** for examples). Ideally, a similar volume of crystalloids should be administered to the donor to replace blood harvested and donors allowed to rest three weeks prior to subsequent collection.

Commercial blood collection kits generally have large-bore 14- to 16-g collection needles attached to the set; however, it is recommended to place a jugular catheter to enable adequate blood collection and for administration of replacement crystalloids, if necessary. Placement of jugular catheters should be aseptic, which requires clipping the hair or wool over the jugular vein and preparing the area with surgical scrub and alcohol. A small amount of lidocaine placed subcutaneously over the vein is useful to minimize movement, especially when performing a stab incision with a scalpel blade. The skin of cows, goats, llamas, and alpacas can be deceptively thick and can create drag on the catheter. A stab incision will reduce drag and facilitate proper placement. Camelid jugular veins are very superficial with prominent valves and are in very close proximity to the carotid artery. It is not uncommon to inadvertently pass through the jugular when placing a catheter and collect an arterial blood sample. If this happens, place pressure with gauze over the puncture site and remove the catheter, holding off for a few minutes before trying again.[33]

The collection kit can be attached to the catheter through an injection port, and the blood can be collected via gravity flow. Agitate or rock the blood bag every few minutes to ensure adequate mixing of anticoagulant and blood. Use of a scale to weigh blood will be more accurate than a visual estimate of volume.

Anticoagulants

The most common anticoagulants for veterinary blood collection include sodium citrate, acid (or anticoagulant) citrate dextrose (ACD), citrate phosphate dextrose (CPD), and heparin.[3]

Table 2
Estimated blood volume of ruminants and corresponding donor volumes to be safely collected at one time

Species	Body Weight (kg)	Total Blood Volume (L)	Blood Volume Safely Harvested (L)
Cow	500	40	8
Sheep/Goat	50	4	0.8
Llama	150	12	2.4

Sodium citrate should only be used when performing an immediate transfusion, because it is metabolized and excreted quickly. It functions as an anticoagulant by chelating calcium and, therefore, should not be mixed with any fluids containing calcium.[3] A 3.85% solution (38.5 g crystalline powder in 1 L sterile water) can be used effectively as an anticoagulant at 100 mL sodium citrate per 1 L blood. Solutions can be autoclaved for sterile administration.[3,4,12,13] Heparin can be used at a dilution rate of 5000 units/L whole blood, or 5 units/mL.[12] In field situations, connect an intravenous administration set to a 1-L bag of isotonic saline, and drain all but 25 to 50 mL and add 5000 units of heparin. Aseptically prepare the jugular for venipuncture and collect 1 L blood through gravity flow.[33] Similar to sodium citrate, heparinized blood should be used for immediate transfusions. Furthermore, use of heparin is contraindicated in cases of on-going hemorrhage or thrombocytopenia, because blood loss will continue because of the prolonged effects of this anticoagulant (plasma half-life of 2 hours).[12]

For collection of blood for storage, ACD is preferred over sodium citrate or heparin. It can be purchased as a sterile, filtered solution in large 500-mL volumes (Anticoagulant Citrate Dextrose Solution USP [ACD] Formula A; Fenwal Inc, Lake Zurich, IL, USA), 50-mL volumes (Sigma-Aldrich, St. Louis, MO, USA), or 25-mL volumes (ACD Solution A; G-Biosciences/Geno Technology Inc, St. Louis, MO, USA). It can also be prepared with the following recipe: 1.8 g (3.6 mL) 50% dextrose solution, 1.6 g sodium citrate, and 0.5 g citric acid. This mixture is dissolved in distilled water to make a total volume of 50 mL.[3] This volume is enough to collect 450 mL blood. For larger volumes of this solution (sufficient for the collection of 6 L blood), 10 g (20 mL) 50% dextrose, 7 g sodium citrate, 8 g citric acid, and distilled water are combined to make a total volume of 1 L.[34] This solution can be autoclaved and decanted as necessary.

Many commercial kits contain CPD or citrate phosphate dextrose adenine-1 (CPDA-1) and a RBC preservative like Optisol (Teruflex blood bag system; Terumo Corporation, Tokyo, Japan). Dextrose provides an energy substrate for ATP production through glycolysis. Phosphate maintains appropriate pH balance for RBC survival and is a substrate to maintain 2,3-diphosphoglycerate (DPG) levels. Maintaining 2,3-DPG levels is important to maximize the release of oxygen from hemoglobin to tissues. In nonruminant species, a low level of 2,3-DPG can indicate reduced erythrocyte survival after transfusion; however, other factors such as chloride and inorganic phosphate seem to modulate oxygen transport out of the bovine erythrocytes.[3,35,36] The Optisol solution is usually for pRBC fractions and contains sodium chloride, dextrose, mannitol, and adenine, which helps stabilize erythrocytes and prevent oxidative damage to cell membranes.[37]

Box 1 shows the equipment recommended for whole blood collection.

Commercial blood collection kits

Plastic collection kits can be obtained from several sources in a variety of sizes, with or without anticoagulant. A 450-mL collection bag would be appropriate for a small ruminant (**Fig. 2**) and 1- to 4-L sized bags for bovine blood collection (Baxter All-In-One Container, Three Lead Transfer Set; Baxter Animal Healthcare Corporation, Deerfield, IL, USA; J-520F Blood Bag, 4L; Jorgensen Laboratories Inc, Loveland, CO, USA). No vacuum exists in the plastic bag collection bags and blood collection must be facilitated through the flow of gravity. Extension sets flushed with anticoagulant should be used when collecting blood in multiple bags.

Commercial blood collection bags that are also used for component separation (Teruflex blood bag system; Terumo Corporation) have a main bag with 63 mL CPD anticoagulant that can hold up to 450 mL blood with a satellite bag containing

---

Box 1
Equipment recommended for whole blood collection

- Adequate restraint (head lock, halter, ± sedation)

- Clippers

- Gauze with surgical scrub (chlorhexidine or iodine) and alcohol

- Lidocaine (1.5–2.0 mL for cattle; 0.5–1.0 mL for sheep/goats)

- 3-cc syringe and 22 to 25-g needles

- Scalpel blade (no. 15)

- Gloves (sterile is preferable)

- Jugular catheter[a] (10–12 g 3.00 inch for bovine; 14–16 g 3.25 inch for sheep/goats/camelids)

- Short extension set with 3-way stopcock[b] and male adapter plugs

- Suture for securing catheter (swaged or premade needles)

- Heparinized flush

- Commercial collection bags[c] or 1- to 2-L collection bags with sufficient anticoagulant and lines flushed before collection

- Gram scale

- Permanent marker

[a] BD Angiocath; Becton Dickinson and Company, Franklin Lakes, NJ.
[b] Smiths Medical ASD, Inc, Dublin, OH.
[c] Teruflex blood bag system; Terumo Corporation.

---

100 mL Optisol Red Cell Preservative solution for pRBCs and empty bags for plasma separation. Care must be taken to collect a specified amount of blood to maintain the correct proportion of anticoagulant and cell preservative to blood volume to prevent red cell damage or excessive anticoagulation within the recipient.

Plastic collection bags or containers are considered preferable for blood collection because it improves RBC storage by reducing hemolysis and decreased clotting factor activation and destruction.[29] Blood collection into glass vacuum bottles (Vacuum Collection Unit, Glass Container; Baxter Healthcare) affects platelets and clotting factors and is not suitable for recipients with on-going hemorrhage or clotting defects.[3,4] For larger volumes required for cattle transfusions, sterile 1- to 4-L plastic blood collection bags can be used with sufficient quantities of desired anticoagulant as described above.

Storage

Storage of units of whole blood can be beneficial, especially in an emergency situation that requires a whole blood transfusion with no immediate access to a donor. However, there are risks associated with storage of whole blood, including changes in red cell shape, decreased flexibility, oxidative stress leading to membrane fragility, and formation of microvesicles, hemolysis, reduced survivability in the recipient's circulatory system, and changes in oxygen delivery and affinity.[3,37] However, some of these red cell lesions are reversible under good storage conditions and rejuvenation occurs with return to normal pH and increased concentrations of ATP.[38] Erythrocytes are dependent on glycolysis for production of energy in the form of ATP along with lactic acid and protons, which reduces the pH of the solution and further inhibits

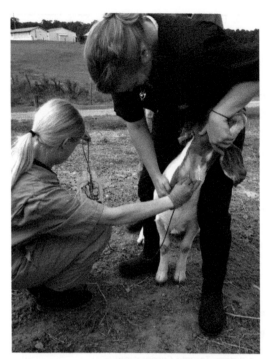

Fig. 2. Field collection from a Boer doe into a commercially available collection bag (Teruflex blood bag system; Terumo Corporation) using the 16-g needle provided. Placement of a catheter to aid in collection is recommended, especially if adequate restraint is not possible. (*Courtesy of* Nikki Schweizer, College of Veterinary Medicine, North Carolina State University.)

ATP production through inhibition of the enzyme phosphofructokinase. Reduction of temperature slows glycolytic pathways and inhibits the ATP-dependent sodium-potassium pump on the erythrocyte membrane; however, there is a persistent potassium leak into the extracellular fluid at a rate of 1 mEq/d.[37,38] Hemolysis during storage can be due to physical and oxidative damage to erythrocyte membranes. In addition, when leukocytes break down, they release glycosidases, lipases, and proteases, which can damage erythrocytes and cause hemolysis. The combination of the use of plastic collection bags, addition of mannitol to stabilize erythrocyte membranes, and filtration or leukoreduction minimizes erythrocyte damage and prolongs the viability of cells in circulation after storage.[38] Oxidative damage to erythrocyte membranes can cause the formation of oxidized lipids. Microvesicles that are formed act as procoagulant and proinflammatory mediators that increase the risk of thrombosis and transfusion-related acute lung injury.[38]

The following describes guidelines suggested for feline and canine blood storage and presumably can be applied similarly to ruminants.[29] Collection sets containing anticoagulant are considered closed collection systems with minimal risk of bacterial contamination. Blood collected via this system can be stored at 1 to 6°C (33–43°F) for up to 28 days depending on the type of anticoagulant used. Blood collected in bags containing CPD can be stored up to 21 days and bags containing CPDA allow viable cells up to 42 days.[37] Open collection systems include using syringes or empty collection bags with anticoagulant added before collection and carry additional risk of microbial contamination. Blood collected in an open system must be used within 4 hours of collection or within 24 hours of collection if stored in a refrigerator.[29] A study in 1983 by Ganesh and Kamalapur[39] demonstrated that storage of bovine erythrocytes stored in ACD at 4°C for 21 days showed no appreciable difference in hematocrit. However, there were increases in plasma potassium, sodium, and lactic acid and decreases in glucose. As mentioned earlier, newer anticoagulant products contain ingredients to reduce hemolysis and storage lesions.

Administration

Box 2 shows the equipment recommended for whole blood administration.

Transfusion recipients should be prepared with a sterile jugular catheter. Care should be taken to not overly stress the patient during this process. As the blood is administered, however, movement should be restricted with panels or straw bales because the animal may move around more and could tangle fluid lines.

Whole blood should be administered via a blood filter (LifeShield Blood Set; Hospira, Inc, Lake Forest, IL, USA; or Fenwal Blood Set; Baxter Health Care) to remove fibrin and microaggregates from the transfused blood (**Fig. 3**). It is helpful to administer isotonic crystalloid fluids that do not contain calcium (0.9% sodium chloride or plasmalyte) to bolus fluids in hypovolemic patients or while in preparation of transfusion. The initial rate of transfusion should be 1 to 5 mL/kg/h for the first 20 minutes, monitoring cardinal signs as frequently as every 2 minutes to observe for evidence of transfusion reactions. After this period, the administration can be increased up to 10 to 20 mL/kg/h, monitoring periodically. Having a multiple port stopcock is useful for administration of 2 separate fluids and as a safety valve in the event of air entering the line. When administering blood from different donors to one recipient, it is recommended to use a separate blood filtration set for each bag, as the blood can clot on

---

Box 2
Equipment recommended for whole blood administration

- Adequate restraint (head lock, halter, ± sedation)
- Clippers
- Gauze with surgical scrub (chlorhexidine or iodine) and alcohol
- Lidocaine (1.5–2.0 mL for bovine; 0.5–1.0 mL for sheep/goats)
- 3-cc syringe and 22- to 25-g needles
- Scalpel blade (no. 15)
- Jugular catheter[a] (bovine: 14–16 g 3.25–5.25 inches; sheep/goats/camelids: 14–16 g 3.25 inch)
- Short extension set with 3-way stopcock[b] and male adapter plugs
- Suture for securing catheter (swaged or premade needles)
- Heparinized flush
- Blood filter administration set[c]
- Crystalloid fluids (0.9% NaCl or Plasmalyte) with administration set
- Thermometer, stethoscope, watch with second hand for monitoring

[a] BD Angiocath; Becton Dickinson and Company.
[b] Smiths Medical ASD, Inc.
[c] LifeShield Blood Set; Hospira Inc; or Fenwal Blood Set; Baxter Health Care.

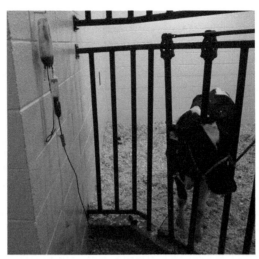

Fig. 3. Holstein steer receiving 450 mL whole blood through a jugular catheter and in-line blood filtration set.

mixing in the lines. The best way to avoid this is to collect as much blood from one donor as possible or use the largest bag size that is appropriate for that patient.

Adverse Reactions

As mentioned earlier, the high variation in blood group factors makes individual blood typing of ruminants impractical and unnecessary, and unlike equine and companion animal medicine, cross-matching via agglutination is not an effective method of determining suitable donor-recipient matches in ruminants. Major cross-matching must be performed with hemolytic testing via complement; however, there may not be sufficient time in an emergency situation.

Adverse reactions to transfusions can be due to cardiovascular overload, erythrocyte incompatibility, and antigenic stimulation from plasma proteins.[3] Typical signs of adverse reactions include tachycardia, tachypnea, shivering, sweating, urticaria, hiccupping, dyspnea, pyrexia, collapse, hypocalcemia, hematuria, hemoglobinuria, and opisthotonus.[3,12,40] Treatment of adverse transfusion reactions involves administration of epinephrine (1:1000) 5 mL intramuscularly (0.01 mg/kg), or 0.5–1.0 mL intravenously (0.001–0.002 mg/kg) in cattle.[12] For goats, a dose of 0.03 mg/kg epinephrine intravenously is recommended for anaphylactic reactions and a similar dose would be expected to be effective in sheep.[11] In the case of urticaria or facial edema, antihistamines such as diphenhydramine at 2 mg/kg intravenously slowly have been reported in canine and feline transfusion reactions.[29] Volume overload can occur in neonatal or pregnant recipients or because of excessive rates of blood or plasma administration, or in endotoxic animals with compromised cardiovascular function.[3] Cardiovascular volume overload can lead to pulmonary hypertension, dyspnea, pulmonary edema, and possibly death. The rate of infusion should be slowed or stopped as soon as clinical signs are observed, and the use of a diuretic, such as furosemide, should be considered as well as oxygen supplementation via nasal insufflation. Hypocalcemia due to citrate toxicity can be mitigated by stopping the transfusion or placing another intravenous catheter and infusing 0.5 to 1.0 mL/kg of 10% calcium gluconate slowly over 10 to 20 minutes, while monitoring the heart rate and rhythm.[29]

BLOOD COMPONENTS
Plasma

Plasma contains immunoglobulins, albumin, coagulation factors (II, VII, IX, X), and additional anti-endotoxic factors. It acts to expand circulating blood volume by increasing colloid osmotic pressure. It can be useful in cases of severe hypoproteinemia and anemia from parasitism, in the event of rodenticide toxicity, and in cases of neonatal FPT. Fresh frozen plasma (FFP) is plasma that has been separated from RBCs within 8 hours of blood collection. It has all the anticoagulants, coagulation factors (labile factors V and VIII; nonlabile factors II, VII, IX, X), albumin, fibrinogen, fibrinonectin, and α-macroglobulin and can be stored at $-40°C$ for 1 year.[41] Frozen plasma is plasma that was been separated from RBCs greater than 8 hours after blood collection, or FFP, which has been stored greater than 1 year but less than 5 years. Frozen plasma generally contains the Vitamin K-dependent nonlabile coagulation factors, but labile factors and anticoagulant activity can be variable.[42]

Indications

Ruminants have syndesmochorial placentas, preventing the transfer of maternal immunoglobulins in utero. Neonates are born agammaglobulinemic and therefore require ingestion of immunoglobulin-rich maternal colostrum to provide adequate antibodies against infection. Neonatal llama and alpaca crias are also at similar risk for FPT if they receive insufficient quality or quantity of maternal colostrum.[43]

In horses with diarrhea, fresh and FFP transfusions have been used as colloidal fluid therapy, providing maintenance of plasma oncotic pressure, clotting factors, and cofactors, and can be presumed to have similar effects in ruminant species.[44] In small animal emergency medicine, plasma products are used in on-going hemorrhage and clotting factor disorders.[42] Plasma transfusions can also be valuable in the treatment of salmonellosis, parasitism, diffuse peritonitis, and warfarin toxicity.[3] The high cost of transfusion and high volumes required to appreciate an increase in total plasma protein concentration may be a limiting factor in the treatment of livestock species; however, it may be useful therapy for valuable calves or small ruminants.

Testing

In general, severe hypoproteinemia can be considered when total plasma proteins are less than 3.0 g/dL and serum albumin is less than 1.5 g/dL, increasing the risk of pulmonary edema and respiratory compromise.[3] FPT can be determined in a variety of ways including history and clinical signs; however, the most common technique involves the measurement of serum total protein concentration by refractometry. Plasma is collected from calves between 24 and 48 hours of birth and levels less than 5.2 g/dL indicate FPT.[45,46] Radial immunodiffusion disk testing is a way to measure serum IgG concentrations and can be performed via commercial kits (Kent Laboratories, Triple J Farms, Bellingham, WA, USA), but takes 24 hours to get results. IgG concentrations less than 1000 mg/dL indicate FPT. Neonatal alpacas and llamas are similar to calves and should be tested around 36 hours for the most accurate total protein or serum IgG concentrations.[43]

Benefits

It is common practice to supplement neonatal foals and camelids that have FPT with FFP transfusions.[47,48] Calves with FPT are at risk of higher mortality in the first few months of life, and thus, supplementation via plasma transfusion has been recommended as a protective treatment.[45,49–51] It has been reported that 1 unit (500 mL) of commercially obtained FFP may be inadequate to sufficiently raise serum IgG levels in FPT calves, and instead a volume of 1.0–1.5 L should be used, depending on calf size and clinical presentation.[52]

When used in cases of systemic inflammatory disease, such as diarrhea, endotoxemia, or septicemia, the benefits include cardiovascular support as well as supplying clotting factors and antioxidant properties.[4] Although it is reported for use in small animal medicine for coagulopathies such as rodenticide toxicity, sepsis, neoplasia, disseminated intravascular coagulopathy, or hepatic failure, there is some variation in opinions regarding the use of plasma products in both human and veterinary medicine.[4,53–55] One study using FFP in canine patients at a rate of 15 to 18 mL/kg did not significantly alter the albumin concentration[55]; however, a rate of 22.5 mL/kg can raise albumin levels by 0.5 g/dL, presuming no on-going protein losses.[42]

Collection technique and commercial sources
There are commercial laboratories that supply veterinary plasma products; however, practitioners need to be sure that the plasma products available are transfusion grade and not intended for research. Many universities have blood donor animals on campus and can have fresh or frozen plasma available for patients, and companies such as Animal Blood Resources Inc (Stockbridge, MI, USA) or Blue Ridge Veterinary Blood Bank (Purcellville, VA, USA) may be able to provide bovine, ovine, caprine, and camelid plasma products if requested. Llama plasma can be ordered from Kent Laboratories, Triple J Farms for use in either llamas or alpacas.

If blood collection kits as described above are used, fresh plasma can be generated through centrifugation and separation into attached satellite bags. Approximately 200 to 250 mL fresh plasma can be obtained from 450 mL whole blood. The bag containing whole blood must be centrifuged at 4°C at 4000 rpm for 10 minutes, transferring the plasma into the satellite plasma bag; the tubing must be cut and tied to maintain sterility and frozen at −20°C for up to 5 years (providing there is no temperature variation).

Plasma separation via plasmapheresis has been reported in equine transfusion medicine.[56] This technique allows larger volumes of plasma to be collected and RBCs to be autotransfused to the donor with the volume of plasma replaced using isotonic crystalloid fluids. The benefits of plasmapheresis include the collection of larger volumes and reduction of cellular components, which may reduce cellular antigens and reduce transfusion actions.[56,57] Some commercial laboratories and universities use this technique for plasma collection and storage.[3]

Technique
It is estimated that a 50-kg foal with complete FPT requires 2 to 4 L plasma to raise IgG levels to between 400 and 800 mg/dL.[47] Plasma transfusion of 20 to 40 mL/kg has been described to be adequate for calves, which would be approximately 1 to 2 L plasma for a 50-kg calf. Chigerwe and Tyler[52] demonstrated that transfusion of 500 mL (1 unit) plasma was insufficient to adequately increase IgG levels in more than 82% of transfused calves. Septic neonates may also require larger volumes or more frequent transfusions because they have greater endothelial permeability and increased utilization of immunoglobulins.[45] Frozen bags of plasma must be handled very carefully, as the plastic becomes very brittle. They are best thawed in a warm water bath, no warmer than body temperature, to reduce damage to the plasma proteins. Plasma should be administered through an intravenous catheter with an appropriate blood filter to remove fibrin or cellular amalgamations, similar to administration of whole blood. Premedication with 1 mg/kg flunixin intravenously before transfusion has been recommended in neonatal camelids.[48] Administration should

be slow, 0.5 mL/kg over the first 10 to 20 minutes and then at a rate of 10 to 40 mL/kg/h.[45] If other intravenous fluids are being administered concurrently; care should be taken not to cause fluid overload by monitoring the flow rate and total volume delivered.

Adverse reactions

Adverse reactions are similar to those described for whole blood transfusion primarily due to fluid overload or allergic reactions with animals exhibiting tachypnea, tachycardia, shivering, and abnormal vocalization.[3,52] Calves, lambs, kids, and crias are particularly susceptible to cardiovascular overload, especially if compromised by systemic illness. Neonatal alpacas receiving a plasma transfusion at a rate of 20 mL/kg/h experienced a reduction in respiratory function, which may be of concern in patients with pre-existing cardiac or pulmonary compromise.[58] Thus, it is extremely important to perform a thorough examination on all animals before transfusion. Adverse effects are usually mild and can be reduced by premedication with nonsteroidal anti-inflammatory drugs or slowing the rate of administration.

Fractionated Blood Products

pRBC

pRBCs remain after centrifugation and removal of plasma from whole blood. They contain mainly RBCs, but possibly also white blood cells unless leukoreduction has taken place.[42] Transfusion of pRBC is indicated in anemia, especially in normovolemic patients (normal total protein) with a nonregenerative process (eg, aplastic anemia or lack of erythropoietin) or hemolytic disease. This component therapy can be especially useful in neonates or patients with cardiovascular compromise with a higher risk of fluid overload, or to provide oxygen-carrying capacity with a smaller volume.[4,42] Calculate the volume of pRBC required with the same calculation used as for whole blood transfusions. As with all other transfusions, it is best performed aseptically with an intravenous catheter, starting with a conservative rate and watching for the adverse reactions mentioned previously.

PRP

PRP is generated from a soft spin (lower centrifugation speed) of whole blood to separate platelets into the plasma component, which is then separated into a separate collection bag. Platelet concentrate can also be generated through automated plateletpheresis techniques to obtain blood components from a donor, as well as other techniques used in human medicine and to some extent in small animal transfusion medicine.[42] PRP transfusion may be indicated in patients with clinical signs of thrombocytopenia, such as petechiae of mucous membranes, spontaneous hemorrhage, or other signs of critical bleeding, such as prolonged epistaxis, hematemesis, and hematochezia.[59] The platelet "transfusion trigger" in canine and feline medicine is considered when signs of any of the above are present, with a platelet count less than 10,000/μL or prophylactic transfusion can be considered in patients undergoing surgery with a platelet count less than 50,000/μL.[59] One unit of PRP is considered the fraction separated from 500 mL whole blood, and a rule of thumb is to transfuse 1 unit/10 kg body weight.[42] In thrombocytopenia, transfusions of fresh whole blood are preferred, due to loss of platelets in the centrifugation process as refrigeration of human plasma results in activation and aggregation of platelets and the reduction of survival time by 50%.[60] Fresh whole blood can be transfused at a rate of 10 mL/kg to raise the platelet count by 10,000/μL, while also providing other clotting factors and components that may be beneficial.[4,42]

Hyperimmune serum

In the most recent *Compendium of Veterinary Products*, there are a few hyperimmune serum products labeled for use in ruminants, primarily of equine origin.[61] The hyperimmune serum products have been reported to enhance colostral absorption of IgG in calves and to be partially protective in piglets against experimental infection of *Haemophilus parasuis*.[62,63] There is minimal research published on the efficacy or safety of the various products on the market mainly aimed at protection against *Escherichia coli*, *Trueperella (formerly Arcanobacterium) pyogenes*, *Pasteurella* spp, and *Clostridium perfringens* type C and D. These products are labeled for calves and lambs via subcutaneous injection or oral administration.

Synthetic Blood Products

In human transfusion medicine, after the 1980s, there was a large demand for an ideal transfusion product that would provide rapid expansion of blood volume, carry oxygen, be available for immediate use, did not require special storage conditions, and did not require blood typing or cross-matching.[64] In 1999, the only licensed polymerized hemoglobin product labeled for veterinary use was Oxyglobin Solution (Bovine hemoglobin glutamer-200 (Formerly Biopure Corporation); OPK Biotech, LLC, Cambridge, MA, USA), which was approved by the United States Food and Drug Administration for the treatment of anemia in dogs. The use of this product was reported in other species including sheep, alpacas, and horses.[65–68] In these case reports, dose rates were conservative, less than the 10 to 30 mL/kg manufacturer recommendation, and the price was often described as a limiting factor. The product was withdrawn from the market in 2010 when Biopure Corporation was purchased by OPK Biotech, LLC. As of February 2013, manufacturing of Oxyglobin has resumed and is being marketed in the European Union by Dechra Veterinary Products. More information can be obtained from their Web site (www.dechra.co.uk). Adverse effects have been described in detail previously and include mucous membrane discoloration, cardiovascular, respiratory, and gastrointestinal effects.[3] If it returns to the American market, it may be a good product for emergency transfusion in valuable neonates, or small ruminant companion animals.

SUMMARY

In conclusion, transfusions of either whole blood or blood components are warranted under certain conditions in ruminant species, and similar to small animal or equine medicine, can be achieved practically both in the hospital and under field situations. Hemolytic or hemorrhagic causes can be indications for whole blood transfusions from infectious or traumatic events. It is important to take a holistic approach when deciding to administer a transfusion of whole blood or whole blood products. The clinical presentation of the patient, as well as the likelihood of response to treatment, availability of a blood donor or transfusion products, are all important factors to determine the success of treatment. Because there is high variability among blood groups and types among ruminant species, a single unmatched transfusion is generally safe. However, the recipient should be monitored for adverse effects. Any subsequent transfusions should have cross-matching performed. Camelids can safely receive either llama or alpaca blood and blood component transfusions. Component transfusions are indicated in certain situations, such as FFP in hypoproteinemia, or pRBCs in normovolemic anemia, but it is important to note that if these components are unavailable, fresh whole blood can be used. Commercial products can be obtained from blood banks for whole blood and blood products, but can also be created in practice, if necessary.

REFERENCES

1. Feldman BF, Joseph ZJ, Jain NC, editors. Schalm's veterinary hematology. 5th edition. Ames (IA): Lippincott, Williams and Wilkins; 2000.
2. Foster A, Bidewell C, Barnett J, et al. Haematology and biochemistry in alpacas and llamas. In Pract 2009;31(6):276–81.
3. Hunt E, Moore JS. Use of blood and blood products. Vet Clin North Am Food Anim Pract 1990;6(1):133–47.
4. Divers TJ. Blood component transfusions. Vet Clin North Am Food Anim Pract 2005;21(3):615–22.
5. Gutierrez G, Reines HD, Wulf-Gutierrez ME. Clinical review: hemorrhagic shock. Crit Care 2004;8(5):373–81.
6. Lelubre C, Vincent JL. Red blood cell transfusion in the critically ill patient. Ann Intensive Care 2011;1:43.
7. van de Watering L. Red cell storage and prognosis. Vox Sang 2011;100(1): 36–45.
8. Smith JE, Dever M, Smith J, et al. Post-transfusion survival of 50Cr-labeled erythrocytes in neonatal foals. J Vet Intern Med 1992;6(3):183–5.
9. Mudge MC, Walker NJ, Borjesson DL, et al. Post-transfusion survival of biotin-labeled allogeneic RBCs in adult horses. Vet Clin Pathol 2012;41(1):56–62.
10. Schnappauf HP, Di Giacomo R, Cronkite EP. Survival of transfused homologous erythrocytes in cattle. Am J Vet Res 1965;26(114):1212–4.
11. Smith MC, Sherman DM. Blood, lymph, and immune systems. In: Smith MC, editor. Goat medicine. Ames (IA): Wiley-Blackwell; 2009. p. 257–338.
12. Soldan A. Blood transfusions in cattle. In Pract 1999;21(10):590–5.
13. Bell G. Blood transfusions in cattle. UK Vet Livestock 2006;11(3):39–43.
14. Rasmusen BA. Blood groups in sheep. Ann N Y Acad Sci 1962;97:306–19.
15. Stormont C. Current status of blood groups in cattle. Ann N Y Acad Sci 1962;97: 251–68.
16. Stormont CJ. Blood groups in animals. J Am Vet Med Assoc 1982;181(10): 1120–4.
17. Blott SC, Williams JL, Haley CS. Genetic relationships among European cattle breeds. Anim Genet 1998;29(4):273–82.
18. Penedo MC. Red blood cell antigens and blood groups in the cow, pig, sheep, goat, and llama. In: Bernard FF, Joseph GZ, Jain NC, editors. Schalm's veterinary hematology. 5th edition. Ames (IA): Lippincott, Williams and Wilkins; 2000. p. 777–82.
19. Hunter N, Foster J, Chong A, et al. Transmission of prion diseases by blood transfusion. J Gen Virol 2002;83(Pt 11):2897–905.
20. Siso S, Gonzalez L, Houston F, et al. The neuropathologic phenotype of experimental ovine BSE is maintained after blood transfusion. Blood 2006;108(2): 745–8.
21. Houston F, McCutcheon S, Goldmann W, et al. Prion diseases are efficiently transmitted by blood transfusion in sheep. Blood 2008;112(12):4739–45.
22. Siso S, Jeffrey M, Houston F, et al. Pathological phenotype of sheep scrapie after blood transfusion. J Comp Pathol 2010;142(1):27–35.
23. McCutcheon S, Alejo Blanco AR, Houston EF, et al. All clinically-relevant blood components transmit prion disease following a single blood transfusion: a sheep model of vCJD. PLoS One 2011;6(8):e23169.
24. Dassanayake RP, Schneider DA, Herrmann-Hoesing LM, et al. Cell-surface expression of PrPC and the presence of scrapie prions in the blood of goats. J Gen Virol 2012;93(Pt 5):1127–31.

25. Dassanayake RP, Schneider DA, Truscott TC, et al. Classical scrapie prions in ovine blood are associated with B lymphocytes and platelet-rich plasma. BMC Vet Res 2011;7:75.
26. Andreoletti O, Litaise C, Simmons H, et al. Highly efficient prion transmission by blood transfusion. PLoS Pathog 2012;8(6):e1002782.
27. Terry LA, Howells L, Bishop K, et al. Detection of prions in the faeces of sheep naturally infected with classical scrapie. Vet Res 2011;42(1):65.
28. Anonymous. National scrapie eradication program. November 2013 Monthly Report. Fiscal Year 2014. Available at: http://www.aphis.usda.gov/animal_health/animal_diseases/scrapie/downloads/monthly_scrapie_rpt.pdf. Accessed May 1, 2014.
29. Gibson G, Abrams-Ogg A. Canine transfusion medicine. In: Day M, Kohn B, editors. BSAVA Manual of Canine and Feline Haematology and Transfusion Medicine. Gloucester (UK): British Small Animal Veterinary Association; 2012. p. 289–307.
30. Waguespack R, Belknap J, Williams A. Laparoscopic management of postcastration haemorrhage in a horse. Equine Vet J 2001;33(5):510–3.
31. Malikides N, Hodgson JL, Rose RJ, et al. Cardiovascular, haematological and biochemical responses after large volume blood collection in horses. Vet J 2001;162(1):44–55.
32. Mudge MC. Blood transfusion in large animals. In: Weiss DJ, Wardrop KJ, editors. Schalm's veterinary hematology. 6th edition. Philadelphia: Lippincott Williams and Wilkins; 2010. p. 757–62.
33. Callan RJ. Small ruminant and camelid critical care tips and tricks. Paper presented at: American Association of Bovine Practitioners. Charlotte, September 25–27, 2008.
34. Eicker SW, Ainsworth DM. Equine plasma banking: collection by exsanguination. J Am Vet Med Assoc 1984;185(7):772–4.
35. Cambier C, Detry B, Beerens D, et al. Effects of hyperchloremia on blood oxygen binding in healthy calves. J Appl Physiol 1998;85(4):1267–72.
36. Gustin P, Detry B, Cao ML, et al. Chloride and inorganic phosphate modulate binding of oxygen to bovine red blood cells. J Appl Physiol 1994;77(1):202–8.
37. Edelstein SB. Blood product storage: does age really matter? Semin Cardiothorac Vasc Anesth 2012;16(3):160–5.
38. Hess JR. Red cell storage. J Proteomics 2010;73(3):368–73.
39. Ganesh T, Kamalapur PN. Biological alterations in bovine blood stored in acid citrate dextrose (ACD) at 4 degrees Celsius. Indian Vet J 1983;60(6):439–44.
40. Radostits OM, Gay CC, Hinchcliff KW, et al. Allergy and anaphylaxis. In: Radostits OM, Gay CC, Hinchcliff KW, et al, editors. Veterinary medicine: a textbook of the diseases of cattle, horses, sheep, pigs and goats. 10th edition. New York: Elsevier Saunders; 2007. p. 70–1.
41. Wardrop KJ, Brooks MB. Stability of hemostatic proteins in canine fresh frozen plasma units. Vet Clin Pathol 2001;30(2):91–5.
42. Davidow B. Transfusion medicine in small animals. Vet Clin North Am Small Anim Pract 2013;43(4):735–56.
43. Weaver DM, Tyler JW, Marion RS, et al. Evaluation of assays for determination of passive transfer status in neonatal llamas and alpacas. J Am Vet Med Assoc 2000;216(4):559–63.

44. Corley KT. Fluid therapy for horses with gastrointestinal disease. In: Smith BP, editor. Large animal internal medicine. 4th edition. St Louis (MO): Mosby Elsevier; 2009. p. 767–79.

45. Barrington GM, Parish SM. Ruminant immunodeficiency diseases. In: Smith BP, editor. Large animal internal medicine. 4th edition. St Louis (MO): Mosby Elsevier; 2009. p. 1677–81.

46. Foster DM, Smith GW, Sanner TR, et al. Serum IgG and total protein concentrations in dairy calves fed two colostrum replacement products. J Am Vet Med Assoc 2006;229(8):1282–5.

47. Sellon DC, Hines MT, Johnson JR. Equine immunodeficiency disease. In: Smith BP, editor. Large animal internal medicine. 4th edition. St Louis (MO): Mosby Elsevier; 2009. p. 1665–77.

48. Whitehead CE. Management of neonatal llamas and alpacas. Vet Clin North Am Food Anim Pract 2009;25(2):353–66.

49. Tyler JW, Hancock DD, Wiksie SE, et al. Use of serum protein concentration to predict mortality in mixed-source dairy replacement heifers. J Vet Intern Med 1998;12(2):79–83.

50. Virtala AM, Grohn YT, Mechor GD, et al. The effect of maternally derived immunoglobulin G on the risk of respiratory disease in heifers during the first 3 months of life. Prev Vet Med 1999;39(1):25–37.

51. Anderson KL, Hunt EF, Fleming SA. Plasma transfusions in failure of colostral immunoglobulin transfer. Bov Pract 1987;22:129–30.

52. Chigerwe M, Tyler JW. Serum IgG concentrations after intravenous serum transfusion in a randomized clinical trial in dairy calves with inadequate transfer of colostral immunoglobulins. J Vet Intern Med 2010;24(1):231–4.

53. Rozanski E, de Laforcade AM. Transfusion medicine in veterinary emergency and critical care medicine. Clin Tech Small Anim Pract 2004;19(2):83–7.

54. Logan JC, Callan MB, Drew K, et al. Clinical indications for use of fresh frozen plasma in dogs: 74 dogs (October through December 1999). J Am Vet Med Assoc 2001;218(9):1449–55.

55. Snow SJ, Ari Jutkowitz L, Brown AJ. Trends in plasma transfusion at a veterinary teaching hospital: 308 patients (1996-1998 and 2006-2008). J Vet Emerg Crit Care (San Antonio) 2010;20(4):441–5.

56. Mischke R. Plasma transfusion and automated plasmapheresis - possibilities and limitations for veterinary medicine. Vet J 2005;169(1):12–4.

57. Feige K, Ehrat FB, Kastner SB, et al. The effects of automated plasmapheresis on clinical, haematological, biochemical and coagulation variables in horses. Vet J 2005;169(1):102–7.

58. Paxson JA, Cunningham SM, Rush JE, et al. The association of lung function and plasma volume expansion in neonatal alpaca crias following plasma transfusion for failure of passive transfer. J Vet Emerg Crit Care 2008;18(6):601–7.

59. Abrams-Ogg AC. Triggers for prophylactic use of platelet transfusions and optimal platelet dosing in thrombocytopenic dogs and cats. Vet Clin North Am Small Anim Pract 2003;33(6):1401–18.

60. Slichter SJ, Harker LA. Preparation and storage of platelet concentrates. Transfusion 1976;16(1):8–12.

61. Anonymous. Compendium of veterinary products: CVP. 13th edition. Port Huron (MI): North American Compendiums, Inc; 2013. Available at: http://bayerall.naccvp.com/?u=bayer&p=dvm. Accessed September 23, 2013.

62. Pedersen RE, Paulrud CO, Tucker WB. Influence of bovine antiserum (Bo-Bac 2X) injection on colostral immunoglobulin G absorption in neonatal dairy calves. J Dairy Sci 2000;83(12):2829–33.

63. Nedbalcova K, Kucerova Z, Krejci J, et al. Passive immunisation of post-weaned piglets using hyperimmune serum against experimental Haemophilus parasuis infection. Res Vet Sci 2011;91(2):225–9.

64. Winslow RM. New transfusion strategies: red cell substitutes. Annu Rev Med 1999;50:337–53.

65. Posner LP, Moon PF, Bliss SP, et al. Colloid osmotic pressure after hemorrhage and replenishment with Oxyglobin Solution, hetastarch, or whole blood in pregnant sheep. Vet Anaesth Analg 2003;30(1):30–6.

66. Langdon Fielding C. A hemoglobin-based oxygen carrier solution for the treatment of parasite-induced anemia in a Barbados sheep. J Vet Emerg Crit Care 2006;16(1):54–7.

67. Dewitt SF, Bedenice D, Mazan MR. Hemolysis and Heinz body formation associated with ingestion of red maple leaves in two alpacas. J Am Vet Med Assoc 2004;225(4):578–83, 539.

68. Vin R, Bedenice D, Rentko VT, et al. The use of ultrapurified bovine hemoglobin solution in the treatment of two cases of presumed red maple toxicosis in a miniature horse and a pony. J Vet Emerg Crit Care 2002;12(3):169–75.

Index

Note: Page numbers of article titles are in **boldface** type.

Vet Clin Food Anim 30 (2014) 475–485
http://dx.doi.org/10.1016/S0749-0720(14)00042-5
0749-0720/14/$ – see front matter © 2014 Elsevier Inc. All rights reserved.

vetfood.theclinics.com

Moving?